ESSENTIALS

LEARNING DISABILITIES

A non-specialist introduction for nursing, health and social care

CHRIS BARBER

Lantern

ISBN: 9781914962004

This book is an updated and revised version of *Caring for People with Learning Disabilities: a guide for non-specialist nurses* published by Lantern Publishing Ltd in 2015 (ISBN 9781908625281)

Lantern Publishing Ltd, The Old Hayloft, Vantage Business Park, Bloxham Rd, Banbury OX16 9UX, UK
www.lanternpublishing.com

British Library Cataloguing in Publication Data
A catalogue record for this book is available from the British Library

The author and publisher have made every attempt to ensure the content of this book is up to date and accurate. However, healthcare knowledge and information is changing all the time so the reader is advised to double-check any information in this text on drug usage, treatment procedures, the use of equipment, etc. to confirm that it complies with the latest safety recommendations, standards of practice and legislation, as well as local Trust policies and procedures. Students are advised to check with their tutor and/or practice supervisor before carrying out any of the procedures in this textbook.

Cover design by AM Graphic Design Ltd
Cover photo by Steve Johnson on Unsplash
Typeset by Medlar Publishing Solutions Pvt Ltd, India
Printed in the UK by Ashford Colour Press Ltd
Last digit is the print number: 10 9 8 7 6 5 4 3 2

Contents

Foreword

Whilst much remains to be achieved to ensure that people with learning disabilities are fully included in society and enjoy full rights to citizenship, there have been many positive developments over recent decades. For example, over the course of my career I have seen the move from predominantly institutional service provision to more community-based forms of support. What has become very evident, however, is that people with learning disabilities continue to experience many inequalities and inequities in relation to health and healthcare. Furthermore, it is clear that to address such disparities is not just the remit of specialist learning disability services: all those working across the range of health and social care provision have a role to play.

However, if this wider responsibility is to be accepted by all health and social care practitioners it is essential that they feel confident and competent to take on this role. Of concern is that a focus on the needs of people with learning disabilities is often not adequately incorporated into the preparation of many health and social care practitioners. Consequently, they may find themselves in a situation where they lack (or feel that they lack) the knowledge and skills required to recognise and appropriately respond to the needs of people with learning disabilities. This, in turn, means that people with learning disabilities may not always receive appropriate support and they continue to experience inequitable access to healthcare.

Of course, it is important that knowledge and skills are developed through direct experience of working alongside and supporting people with learning disabilities. However, this book seeks to provide students and practitioners with the foundational knowledge they need to deliver effective support and thus increase their confidence when giving such support.

As noted above, services and supports for people with learning disabilities continue to evolve, as do our knowledge and understanding. An updated version of this book is therefore to be welcomed since it has been revised to take account of recent developments that impact on the lives of people with learning disabilities and their families. It provides not just knowledge but also aims to assist you with applying this knowledge to your practice through scenarios and reflective activities.

The closing sentences of the final chapter in this book challenge you to become a power for positive change in the lives of people with learning disabilities: a failure to do so risks them continuing to experience disparities in health and wellbeing that are avoidable. I hope, therefore, that you will not only read this volume but that you will also reflect upon how you can make a positive contribution. Do not feel that any changes you make are insignificant – if everyone working in health and social care made small positive changes in practice this would add up to wide-scale change for people with learning disabilities.

Ruth Northway (OBE, FRCN, PFHEA)
Professor of Learning Disability Nursing
University of South Wales

Preface

If you ever engage with a person with a learning disability, either in hospital, at a GP practice, in a community setting or even in the person's own home and wonder: How do I find out and understand what this person's needs are? How can I provide the best possible care for this person? Well, you are not alone and this book is definitely for you. So, welcome!

The world has changed since 2015 when the first edition of this book was published (with the title *Caring for People with Learning Disabilities*) and this current book was intended to be an updated second edition. Since being 'invited' to write this new edition which takes a whole lifetime approach (from birth to death) and covers most areas of care that the person with a learning disability is likely to need during that timeframe, the book has taken on a life of its own. It has broken free from the 'shackles' imposed by being a mere updated version of the first edition. It has become a living and breathing entity in its own right!

So, sit back and enjoy this book and if, in the process of reading it, you find something that you did not previously know and that you can use in your work as a nurse or health and social care worker when working with a person with a learning disability, then great! The book has done its job!

Chris Barber

Acknowledgements

I would like to thank my late wife Jean, who very sadly passed away during the writing of this second edition, and my son Freddie for their support and patience during the writing of this book.

Furthermore, I would like to thank the reviewers for their kind and thoughtful comments and suggestions regarding the text.

Finally, I would like to thank Mark Allen Publishing for their kind permission to reproduce text that was first published by the *British Journal of Healthcare Assistants*.

This book is dedicated to Jean. May she rest in peace.

About the author

The author is a registered nurse (learning disabilities), qualifying as such in December 1989. He has worked in a wide variety of clinical settings, both residential and community, with a wide variety of service users (those who are on the autism spectrum, those with sensory impairments, those whose behaviour 'challenges services', those who require forensic services and care and those with mental health issues). He is a parent of a young man who is also on the autism spectrum and he himself was diagnosed at the end of 2008 as being 'high-functioning autistic'. He holds an MEd from the University of Birmingham in special educational needs (autism). He sits on the editorial board of the *British Journal of Nursing*, the *British Journal of Healthcare Assistants* and the *British Journal of Mental Health Nursing*, and as well as having written a number of articles / papers on a wide variety of subjects including learning disabilities, caregivers, spirituality and autism, he is the author of *Autism and Asperger's Conditions*, published by Quay Books. Chris currently works as a visiting lecturer in learning disability nursing at Birmingham City University.

Chapter 1
Introduction

LEARNING OUTCOMES FOR THE BOOK

By the end of this book you will:

1.1 Gain an understanding of and be able to discuss what learning disability is and is not

1.2 Gain an understanding of and be able to discuss a wide range of issues that impact upon the lives of those with a learning disability, from conception to death

1.3 Apply this understanding critically when working with those who have a learning disability

1.4 Apply this understanding critically in order to improve the quality of nursing care that those with a learning disability experience.

1.1 Who is this book for?

This book is intended for those nursing students, staff nurses, nursing associates and healthcare assistants (HCAs) who are not learning disability specialists but who, as a result of working with those who have a learning disability, would like to learn more about and understand learning disability as a condition and hence provide better care and support for those with a learning disability. For ease of reading and to prevent the text from becoming cumbersome, the term 'nurse' is intended to include other healthcare professionals as well.

In 2016 Oliver McGowan, a teenager with autism, died in hospital having been given antipsychotic medication against his and his family's wishes. Following Oliver's death, his mother Paula led a campaign for more training for health and social care staff to provide them with the confidence and skills to understand the needs of people with learning disabilities and/or autism in their care. In 2019, Skills for Care and Skills for Health published an update of the Core Capabilities Framework for Supporting People with a Learning Disability. There is a corresponding Core

Capabilities Framework for Supporting Autistic People (see the *Resources* section at the end of the chapter for links to both the frameworks). A standardised training package is being developed, coordinated by Health Education England and Skills for Care and named after Oliver McGowan (HEE, 2021), which will be mandatory for health and social care staff, at the right level for their role, to provide better health and social care outcomes for people with a learning disability and autistic people.

The core capabilities frameworks describe the skills, knowledge and behaviours that professionals who support people with a learning disability and/or autism are required to bring to their work, and they are set out at three tiers:

Tier 1 – those who require general understanding and awareness of learning disabilities or autism and the support needed by people with a learning disability or autism.

Tier 2 – health and social care professionals with responsibility for providing care and support for people with a learning disability or autism, but who would seek support from other professionals for complex management or complex decision-making.

Tier 3 – health, social care and other professionals with a high degree of autonomy, able to provide care in complex situations and who may also lead services for people with autism or a learning disability.

This book is intended to set you on the road to attaining the core capabilities that you will need and to give you a solid foundation for the mandatory training you will be required to undertake at some stage during your career.

As the following three boxes show, learning disability registered nurses face a number of professional challenges. Consequently, the support that the practitioner who is not a learning disability nurse will be able to offer both to those with a learning disability and to learning disability nurses is likely to become increasingly important.

> "Problems attracting people into learning disability nursing training have 'come to a head' and there is now a risk there will be an insufficient number of new nurses working in this field in the future, the national workforce body has said."
>
> (Merrifield, 2017)

> "A care centre looking after vulnerable patients with disabilities has been branded a site of 'psychological torture' following a three-month undercover report. Sixteen staff in Whorlton Hall in County Durham have been suspended after an investigation by BBC Panorama found staff abusing patients in their care."
>
> (inews, 2019)

"There are continuing concerns regarding the challenges that people with learning disabilities face and the future of learning disability nursing. The decline in the number of learning disability nurses has continued in the five years since the first RCN *Connect for Change* report and we are now seeing 40% fewer learning disability nurses in the NHS in England since May 2010, from 5,368 in May 2010 to 3,217 in July 2020."

(RCN, 2021)

Indeed, given these professional challenges facing many learning disability nurses, it is possible for the non-specialist nurse or healthcare professional to come into their own here and make a significant and positive impact upon the care experienced by those who have a learning disability.

PAUSE FOR THOUGHT 1.1

Ask yourself why you think that having another book on learning disability nursing care and support will improve the care that is experienced by those with a learning disability. What do you hope to gain from this book? Why did you buy it and why are you reading it? Keep a journal of your thoughts and practices as you read this book and ask yourself these questions again once you have finished reading it. Compare and contrast your two sets of answers.

There are a number of books that will be useful in supporting and caring for both adults and children with learning disabilities. Jukes (2009), Peate and Fearns (2006), Clark and Griffiths (2008) and Moulster *et al.* (2019) all spring to mind here. There are also an increasing number of books about autism spectrum conditions that may be of use, including Barber (2011).

The reason for this book is to provide the care professional who is not a learning disability specialist with practical suggestions, which are easy to both follow and implement, for supporting this client group. It is not the intention to replicate the contents of other books but to highlight areas that seem to 'fall between the cracks' and consequently are rarely if ever mentioned within other books: discrimination, spirituality, 'informal caregivers' and sexuality, as well as dying, death and bereavement. This book attempts to present challenging content in a way that stimulates thought and reflection, in order to help you provide better care. It is not meant to suggest that nursing care for those with a learning disability is poor; indeed, far from it! However, there may be occasions when the attitudes and practices of some HCAs, nursing students and registered nurses may need to be challenged. If through the process of this challenging, people have been offended, then apologies are offered, and forgiveness sought.

There are also a large number of journals and journal articles by countless authors about those with a learning disability, the families of those with a learning disability, learning disability nurses and the learning disability care workforce in general. Both the *Nursing Standard* and *Nursing Times* have published a range of online articles on learning disability care, some of which are free to download. However, there still appears to be a real and serious gap in the knowledge of many non-specialist nurses, doctors, social care staff and the professions allied to medicine (PAMS: physiotherapists, occupational therapists and paramedics) regarding the lives and needs of those with a learning disability.

PAUSE FOR THOUGHT 1.2

How much do you *really* know about learning disability and those with a learning disability?

In any given week where you work, how many of your patients or service users do you think have a learning disability?

Is your knowledge of learning disability enough to provide the type and level of care and support that you would like and that your patients or service users need and have a right to?

A lack of knowledge and understanding of learning disability will pose challenges to nurses who are not learning disability specialists but are responsible for the provision of high-quality care, and is likely to have a negative impact on the form and quality of care experienced by those with a learning disability (Mencap, 2007).

As far back as 1979, the Jay Report (Jay Committee, 1979) recommended the ending of learning disability as a nursing branch. Such recommendations have been echoed over many years during debates at RCN Congress.

The Nursing and Midwifery Council (NMC) has in the past tried to restructure pre-registration nurse training with a view to establishing a generalist nurse who would, in theory, have enough knowledge and skills to work in any clinical setting and with any clinical group. Learning disability, mental health and paediatric branches could all be followed at post-registration level. Indeed, such an approach received much, but by no means universal support within nursing's senior management and leadership and was also resisted by many nurses.

But what of the roles of the nurse, nursing student, HCA, physiotherapist, occupational therapist, paramedic or social care worker who is not a learning disability specialist? After all, most of these books that are available on the subject of learning disability and the care and support of those with a learning disability are aimed, primarily, at those working within the field of learning disability care and support. However, all nurses and other health professionals are likely to come into contact and work with people with a learning disability at some point in their careers. Indeed, the NMC standards of proficiency for registered nurses (NMC, 2018a) and standards for education and training (NMC, 2018b) require cross-curricular learning across all fields of nursing practice so that all nurses can meet the person-centred, holistic care needs of the people they encounter in their practice "who may be at any stage of life and who may have a range of mental, physical, cognitive or behavioural health challenges".

Partly to meet this requirement, four fictional but authentic examples of people involved in one way or another in the care of people with learning disabilities will be introduced here and they will appear in case studies throughout the book.

Sally is a senior staff nurse with five years' post-qualifying experience, first in an A&E department and then in an acute medical ward of her local general hospital. Sally says that she occasionally encounters patients who have a learning disability but does not feel confident in meeting their specific care needs.

Hanif is a '40-something' second-year student nurse who is following the 'adult branch'. Before commencing his nurse training, Hanif worked as an HCA in the same A&E department as Sally. Hanif would like to learn more about learning disability than he feels that he currently learns from his training.

Jill is an HCA who has worked at her local GP practice and community health centre for the past six years after working in an office for a year. Jill has a younger sister who has Down's syndrome.

Chris is a registered nurse for those with a learning disability and is the author of this, his second book. Chris, who has Asperger's syndrome / high-functioning autism, currently works as a full-time caregiver for his wife and son and is a visiting lecturer in learning disability nursing at Birmingham City University.

1.2 A brief overview of the book

In order to fill some of these gaps in knowledge and understanding, this short book will focus on a number of issues pertinent to the understanding, care and support of those with a learning disability in a world that has changed over the past decade, a world that will continue to change. The issue of mandatory training and development regarding meeting the person-centred needs of those with a learning disability will be raised and discussed throughout the book: see https:// skillsforhealth.org.uk/info-hub/learning-disability-and-autism-frameworks-2019/

Three further fictional but authentic examples of people with learning disabilities are now introduced here who will also appear in case studies throughout the book.

Marcel is a '30-something' man who was born in Morocco and who happens to have Down's syndrome. He lives at home with his parents who are in their 60s and his pet cat that he calls 'Moggy'. Marcel works part time at the café at his local supermarket. His elder sister, Ziva, is married and has two children. Marcel's hobbies include music, 'Red Dwarf', country walks and meeting people.

Ziva, who is Marcel's sister, has Asperger's syndrome / high-functioning autism. She is married and has two children, one of whom is also on the autism spectrum. Ziva works part time as a university lecturer in pure and applied maths.

Thomas is 65 years old and has a profound and multiple learning disability with additional severe mobility problems, pre-verbal communication skills, inability to digest food, arthritis and epilepsy. Thomas lives within a social care home.

Chapter 2 gives a definition of learning disability. There are a number of definitions and unless one is able to understand what learning disability is, it could be suggested that health and social care and support of those with a learning disability will be impoverished. The lived meaning and experience of having a learning disability will be highlighted through the eyes of Marcel, Ziva and Thomas.

The meaning of profound and multiple learning disability will be focused on in *Chapter 3* and will be informed by the experiences of Thomas.

There have been many government and independent sector reports over the last 50 years or so around the services for, and the quality of life of those with a learning disability. These have included reports about some of the learning disability hospitals such as Ely and South Ockendon hospitals in the early 1970s, the Jay Report in the late 1970s, the White Paper *Valuing People* (DH, 2001), the Mencap report *Death by Indifference* in 2007 and reports about the deaths of a number of people with a learning disability while in NHS care facilities (Mencap 2013, 2014, 2019). *Chapter 4* will focus on and explain what these reports and any subsequent legislation mean for nurses, nursing students, nursing associates, HCAs, social care staff and PAMs working with people with a learning disability.

Many, if not most, healthcare professionals are likely at some point in their work to encounter and provide healthcare support to those with a learning disability. *Chapter 5* will focus on how to provide high quality support within a number of generalist healthcare environments including health centres, GP practices, outpatient departments and acute / medical or surgical wards of a general hospital.

Chapter 6 will focus on the often complex area of consent to treatment and intervention with regard to those with a learning disability. Just because a person has a learning disability does not necessarily mean that they cannot give, withhold or withdraw consent.

Although learning disability and mental ill-health are not the same thing, there is an overlap between the two. *Chapter 7* will focus on the mental health needs of those with a learning disability.

Some of those with a learning disability will commit crimes; occasionally, some of these crimes will be of a very serious nature including assault, murder, sexual assault, rape and arson and will require specialist forensic services. *Chapter 8* will focus on the care and support of those with a learning disability who require such specialist services.

The subject of sexuality, relationships and those with a learning disability as parents has always been very controversial. *Chapter 9* will focus on the sexual and relationship needs of those with a learning disability.

The challenges and delights of ageing for those with a learning disability and those who care for them will be highlighted in *Chapter 10*.

Although learning disability does not necessarily equate to having a short lifespan as once it did, dying and death are part and parcel and the inevitable conclusion of all life, of all humanity. *Chapter 11* will focus on end of life processes and the role of the nurse and HCA in this process.

Many, if not most, people with a learning disability will live at home with their parents and siblings rather than in a non-family residential setting such as a learning disability hospital or community home. *Chapter 12* will focus on the experiences and needs of families who look after a person with a learning disability.

There has been a long and very sad and painful history of discrimination against those with a learning disability and their families. Following on from the previous chapter on the care and support of 'informal caregivers', *Chapter 13* will focus on this history and the role of the nurse, HCA, social care staff and PAMs in combating such discrimination and prejudice.

Spirituality is not about ticking the 'Church of England' box on the service user's assessment form or attention to the cultural and religious dimensions of diet, clothing and personal hygiene. *Chapter 14* will focus on and explore a definition and applicability of spirituality to those with a learning disability.

The final chapter will look back and reflect in order to look forward, with a view to suggesting a small number of future developments in learning disability services and care.

The appendices comprise a brief glossary of learning disability terms and a short selection of resources on learning disability, those with a learning disability and practical suggestions on how to support those with a learning disability.

Ziva, being a university lecturer, may be an odd person to act as a guide in a book about learning disabilities as the inclusion of Asperger's syndrome, or high-functioning autism as it is sometimes known, in the umbrella term of learning disability is debatable. However, Ziva says that she will delve into this issue in the next chapter. On the other hand, being Marcel's sister, she is able to provide much useful information regarding life with a learning disability. The stories of Thomas, Marcel and Ziva will unfold over the coming pages and chapters, but at the moment they would just like to say "Hi"!

All that remains to be said here is welcome to this short book. I hope that you will enjoy reading it, that it will challenge how you think about and interact with those who have a learning disability and that it will be of use and benefit to you in your daily work.

Questions

Question 1.1   What do you hope to gain from this book? Why did you buy it and why are you reading it? You may like to revisit this question once you have finished reading the book.

Question 1.2   Is your knowledge of learning disability enough to provide the type and level of care and support that you would like and that your patients or service users need?

Question 1.3   What help and support do you need to provide good quality care to those with a learning disability?

REFERENCES

Barber, C. (2011) *Autism and Asperger's Conditions: a practical guide for nurses.* Quay Books.

Clark, L. and Griffiths, P. (2008) *Learning Disability and Other Intellectual Impairments.* John Wiley & Sons.

Department of Health (2001) *Valuing People: a new strategy for learning disabilities for the 21st century.* HMSO.

HEE (2021) *The Oliver McGowan Mandatory Training in Learning Disability and Autism.* Available at: www.hee.nhs.uk/our-work/learning-disability/oliver-mcgowan-mandatory-training-learning-disability-autism (accessed 30 December 2021).

inews (2019) *Whorlton Hall: BBC Panorama investigation shows care stuff abusing vulnerable adults in County Durham hospital.* Available at: https://inews.co.uk/news/whorlton-hall-panorama-bbc-county-durham-hospital-abuse-vulnerable-adults-video-294311 (accessed 30 December 2021).

Jay Committee (1979) *The Report of the Committee of Enquiry into Mental Handicap Nursing and Care.* Department of Health / HMSO.

Jukes, M. (ed.) (2009) *Learning Disability Nursing Practice.* Quay Books.

Mencap (2007) *Death by Indifference.* Mencap. Available at: www.mencap.org.uk/sites/default/files/2016-06/DBIreport.pdf (accessed 30 December 2021).

Mencap (2013) *Mencap research: "scandal of avoidable death" as 1,200 people with a learning disability die needlessly every year in NHS care*. Available at: www.mencap.org.uk/press-release/mencap-research-scandal-avoidable-death-1200-people-learning-disability-die (accessed 30 December 2021).

Mencap (2014) *Charities continue fight for justice as young man dies in NHS care*. Available at: www.mencap.org.uk/press-release/charities-continue-fight-justice-young-man-dies-nhs-care (accessed 30 December 2021).

Mencap (2019) *Mencap welcomes the independent review into the death of Oliver McGowan*. Available at: www.mencap.org.uk/press-release/mencap-welcomes-independent-review-death-oliver-mcgowan (accessed 30 December 2021).

Merrifield, N. (2017) Risk of 'insufficient' learning disability nurses being trained. *Nursing Times*. Available at: www.nursingtimes.net/roles/learning-disability-nurses/risk-of-insufficient-learning-disability-nurses-being-trained-18-10-2017 (accessed 30 December 2021).

Moulster, G., Iorizzo, J., Ames, S. and Kernohan, J. (eds) (2019) *The Moulster and Griffiths Learning Disability Nursing Model: a framework for practice*. Jessica Kingsley Publishers.

Nursing and Midwifery Council (2018a) *Future Nurse: Standards of proficiency for registered nurses*. NMC.

Nursing and Midwifery Council (2018b) *Realising Professionalism: Standards for education and training*. NMC.

Peate, I. and Fearns, D. (2006) *Caring for People with Learning Disabilities*. John Wiley & Sons.

Royal College of Nursing (2021) *Connecting for Change: for the future of learning disability nursing*. RCN. Available at: www.rcn.org.uk/professional-development/publications/connecting-for-change-uk-pub-009-467 (accessed 30 December 2021).

RESOURCES

Core Capabilities Framework for Supporting People with a Learning Disability. Available at: https://skillsforhealth.org.uk/wp-content/uploads/2020/11/Learning-Disability-Framework-Oct-2019.pdf (accessed 30 December 2021).

Core Capabilities Framework for Supporting Autistic People. Available at: https://skillsforhealth.org.uk/wp-content/uploads/2020/11/Autism-Capabilities-Framework-Oct-2019.pdf (accessed 30 December 2021).

Chapter 2
What is learning disability?

AIMS AND LEARNING OUTCOMES

The aims of this chapter are to:

2.1 Present and discuss two 'dictionary' type definitions of learning disability

2.2 Highlight and discuss the identity of learning disability.

By the end of this chapter you will be able to:

2.3 Discuss the definition, meaning and identity of learning disability from a range of different standpoints

2.4 Discuss how these definitions, meanings and identities have changed over time

2.5 Discuss how these will continue to change.

SCENARIO 2.1

Marcel, a 39-year-old man with Down's syndrome, is admitted, having had a stroke, onto the general medical ward on which Hanif works as part of a 2nd year student nurse placement. This is the first time that Hanif has had a patient with Down's syndrome and he knows very little about learning disability in general and Down's syndrome in particular. At the handover at the start of Hanif's shift, he asks: 'What is learning disability?'

PAUSE FOR THOUGHT 2.1

A nurse, who during a debate at RCN Congress said that he considers himself to have Asperger's syndrome, was asked: "What is this disease called Asperger's?" Do you, the reader, consider learning disability to be a disease? Do you consider that learning disability is catching? What would be the implications and consequences for the person with a learning disability and the nurse if learning disability is a disease?

2.1 Introduction

What is learning disability? You would be forgiven for asking this question, particularly if you have not previously worked with people who have a learning disability. Following on from this initial question, a number of further questions could be asked: What does it mean to have a learning disability? Indeed, to develop this further, what does it mean to be 'learning disabled'?

A careful reading of the above questions seems to highlight four different issues:
- A need for a basic, clear and factual definition of learning disability
- A need for a discussion around learning disability as possession, in much the same way as having or possessing a broken leg or a broken arm or having a headache
- A need to discuss the validity and appropriateness of using a 'disease model' when thinking about learning disability
- A need for a discussion around learning disability as personal identity.

These are all valid and perfectly reasonable questions to ask, particularly if you have had very little if any previous knowledge or experience of, or exposure to learning disability as either an 'abstract' or a 'physical' concept or reality. Appropriate theoretical learning and clinical experience opportunities around learning disabilities may not always be available to you.

Again, there is a continuing perception that learning disability is a 'childhood' condition; or there may be some confusion as to 'learning disabilities' and 'learning difficulties', with some people thinking that these two terms refer to the same condition or phenomenon. Learning difficulties or specific learning difficulties usually refer to the specific conditions of dyslexia, dyspraxia and dyscalculia. Specific Learning Difficulties (SpLDs) affect the way information is learned and processed. They are neurological (rather than psychological), usually run in families and occur independently of intelligence. They can have significant impact on education and learning and on the acquisition of literacy skills (British Dyslexia Association, undated).

2.2 Definition

What does this term 'learning disability' actually mean?

Barber (2011) suggested that the term 'learning disability' cannot be defined easily. Learning disability can act as a category for a variety of conditions with different causes. Some forms of learning disability are as possible results of:
- 'genetic abnormalities': Down's syndrome, phenylketonuria, Marfan's syndrome and tuberous sclerosis (epiloia) are all examples of genetic causes
- major difficulties during or immediately after childbirth
- alcohol or 'recreational drug' use during pregnancy
- environmental factors such as environmental or industrial toxins.

Other forms of learning disability just are: these are known as 'idiopathic'. An idiopathic (from the Greek *idios* ('one's own') and *pathos* ('suffering')) disease or condition is one whose cause is not known or one that arises spontaneously.

However, it could be argued that these are the causes of learning disability, rather than what learning disability is (and is not).

There are a number of ways of looking at the term 'learning disability' and hence those with a learning disability. The first of these is to focus on learning disability as a 'dictionary definition'. Again, there are a number of such definitions that can be explored. The first of these definitions is taken from the *Valuing People* White Paper (DH, 2001: 14). According to *Valuing People*, a person is described as having a learning disability if they have:

- a significantly reduced ability to understand new or complex information (impaired intelligence and cognitive functioning)
- a significantly reduced ability to learn new skills (impaired intelligence and cognitive functioning), with
- a reduced ability to cope independently (impaired social functioning) and
- which started before adulthood and with a lasting effect on development.

An alternative definition is provided by the Mental Health Act 1983, Section 1:

- An arrested or incomplete development of mind
- that impacts upon most if not all areas of human life: intellectual, spiritual, physical, educational and social
- and ranges in severity and impact from borderline to profound
- with the likelihood of multiple neurological and physical disabilities increasing with serious and profound learning disabilities
- and that often requires additional supportive resources in order to facilitate optimum physical, mental, spiritual, social and emotional health and engagement within society.

However, both of these definitions could be argued to pose a number of questions or problems. First: the Department of Health definition. *Valuing People* was the first learning disability White Paper for nearly a quarter of a century.

> A White Paper is formal Government policy on a given subject such as learning disability, as opposed to a Green Paper which is a discussion or consultation document and a Bill or Act of Parliament. A White Paper has no force of law behind it and cannot, therefore, be enforced in the same way as an Act of Parliament such as the Autism Act 2009.

The definition given in the White Paper is still the 'definition of choice', although the meaning has been 'simplified' by various organisations such as the NHS (2018) and Mencap (undated) and can be found as such in many learning disability textbooks; it is both concise and accurate. However, it lacks in its apparent objectivity and simplicity the possibility that learning disability is not a single condition, but a series of conditions. These conditions range from 'borderline' learning disability through to 'profound' learning disabilities via 'mild', 'moderate' and 'severe' learning disabilities. The more severe the learning disability is, the more likely that such learning disability will include increasing physical disabilities such as cerebral palsy, musculoskeletal issues such as scoliosis, neurological conditions such as epilepsy, sensory issues such as impaired hearing and sight, and medical conditions such as respiratory and cardiac problems.

Again, although succinct and relatively easy to understand, this definition runs the risk of locating the disability within rather than outside the person. The suggestion here is that disability is imposed by societal attitudes and practices which prevent people with a learning disability from fully engaging with society.

Where would one place autism as a learning disability? The classic form of autism involves a triad of impairments relating to social interaction, social communication and the use of language, and limited imagination as reflected in restricted, repetitive and stereotyped patterns of behaviour and activities. Few people would argue that this 'classic autism' is not a form of learning disability, as it shares many of the cognitive issues and impairments of learning disability. However, would people such as Bill Gates (founder of Microsoft), Keith Joseph (British politician, 1918–94), Ludwig Wittgenstein (Austrian philosopher, 1889–1951), Peter Sellers (British comedian, 1925–80), Gary Numan (British electronic musician), Chris Packham (naturalist, conservationist and television presenter) and Anne Hegerty (quiz show personality (*The Chase*)), all of whom are or were suggested to have Asperger's syndrome, fit comfortably within a traditional learning disability framework? Probably not! Again, since those with Asperger's tend to have higher than average IQs, given the names mentioned above, is Asperger's an aspect of learning disability?

The second definition is based on the opening section of the 1983 Mental Health Act and probably comes closest to providing a legal definition of learning disability. However, this definition also applies to those with mental health issues and is not specific to learning disability. Again, the concept of 'mind' is introduced but, sadly, is not defined or developed. Having said that, this definition appears to be more 'holistic' in tone and acknowledges that learning disability is a spectrum of conditions.

Although the connection between IQ levels and levels of learning disability is now seen as outmoded, learning disability has been defined in terms of intelligence quotient (IQ), a scale that was used to measure intellectual or mental ability. In general, IQ levels indicated that (WHO, 2010):

People with an IQ level of	Were classified as
70 and above	'Normal'
50 to 69	'Mild' learning disability
35 to 49	'Moderate' learning disability
20 to 34	'Severe' learning disability
Less than 20	'Profound' learning disability

The general effectiveness of IQ ratings in indicating the level of a person's learning disability is contested as being arbitrary, crude and inaccurate (New Scientist, 2009), and may not therefore be the best method of indicating learning disability.

However, another way of viewing learning disability is to see learning disability as a combination of intellectual and physical or health conditions (Garvey and Vincent, 2006). A practical example of this view would be those with Down's syndrome, who are likely to experience difficulties in a number of different ways. These differences could include:

- communication problems
- a tendency to being overweight
- problems with balance and mobility
- painful joints and muscles
- mental health issues
- sensory issues
- heart problems
- respiratory problems.

There may be other healthcare issues that those with a learning disability may experience. However, it has to be said that not every person with a learning disability will experience all of these health issues. Again, caution must be applied here as many people who do not have a learning disability may also experience some or many of the health issues above, at some point in their lives.

PAUSE FOR THOUGHT 2.2

Now here is a question: how many people in the UK do you think are affected by learning disability?

You would be forgiven if you either plucked a figure randomly out of the air or said that you did not have a clue. You are probably not alone if you gave either of these answers! Estimates of how many people experience learning disabilities vary. For example, according to Public Health England, in 2014/15, 70 065 children in England with a primary need associated with learning disabilities had a statement of special educational needs / education health and care plan. Of these, 44% were identified as having moderate learning difficulties (MLD), 41% severe learning difficulties (SLD) and 15% profound and multiple learning difficulties (PMLD) (PHE, 2016, p. 5). Corresponding data for adults is hard to come by, as some areas of learning disability statistics are not compiled or held centrally by the UK Government (PHE, 2016, p. 10).

However, using data from Public Health England and the Office for National Statistics, Mencap estimates that there are about 1.5 million people in the UK who have a learning disability, made up of about 1 130 000 adults and 351 000 children. For more detail on these figures and references to the data, see the Mencap website at www.mencap.org.uk/learning-disability-explained/research-and-statistics/how-common-learning-disability.

The question asked in *Pause for thought 2.2* was how many people *are affected by* learning disability, not how many people *have* a learning disability. By asking how many people are affected by learning disability, the families, relatives, friends and even care professionals, each with their own expectations, needs and even agendas, must be included. Whilst there are around 1.5 million people in the UK with a learning disability, those *affected* by learning disability will be much higher. It must also be kept in mind that 'learning disability' is not the same as 'learning difficulties', as the latter relates to neurodiverse conditions such as dyslexia, dyscalculia and dysgraphia.

2.3 Basic history

> **PAUSE FOR THOUGHT 2.3**
>
> Student nurses following the learning disability pathway today will, when they qualify, register as 'Registered Nurse (learning disability)'. When I qualified as a learning disability nurse in 1989, my qualification was 'Registered Nurse (mental handicap)'. My tutors' and lecturers' qualification was 'Registered Nurse (mental subnormality)'. In terms of language, where do we go from here?

Why is it important to look at the history of learning disability? After all, it could be suggested that it is where we are now and where we are going that is important!

If you are aware of and understand the history of learning disability, how language has framed the definitions of learning disability and disability discourse over the decades, how such definitions and discourse and how those with a learning disability have been viewed have changed over time, then you may be able to understand the present better. If you understand the present, then you can see how the future might be shaped for the better. To put this observation another way, those who do not have awareness and understanding of the past are condemned to repeat its mistakes! As can be seen from *Pause for thought 2.3*, the history of learning disability and those with a learning disability is bound intimately to language and its use. The lives of those with a learning disability and the ways that they have been treated by society in general, and health and social care professionals in particular, have changed for the better when the language that in part defines them has changed.

Learning disability is not a recent condition by any means; it was likely that learning disability existed in biblical times. It may not have been inconceivable that learning disability, autism spectrum conditions and mental health conditions were considered to be examples of demon possession or a result of sin (Heuser, 2012; Romero, 2012). During the Middle Ages those with learning disabilities were either considered to be the 'village idiot', or due to their simplicity and naivety 'God's holy fools', and either exalted or reviled, feared and hated. Many of those with a learning disability, an autism spectrum condition or a mental health issue would have been considered to be witches due to their behaviour and condemned accordingly. Again, those with a learning disability would likely have been left on the street to either barely survive through begging, to be 'cared for' by the Church or to die. From 1850 to 1910 (Gilbert, 2009) a more 'formalised' approach to care began to emerge which seemed to coincide with changes in social philosophy and policy. Those with a learning disability were seen as harmless but 'sub-human'. The emphasis of service provision was on separation and segregation of those with either a learning disability or mental health issue from the rest of society. However, those with borderline or mild learning disabilities were considered fit for menial, largely rural, work.

The overriding form of care in the first half of the twentieth century for those with a learning disability was the 'colony' (Gilbert, 2009). A 'colony' was a large mental subnormality/mental handicap hospital, usually situated in rural areas. Hospitals such as South Ockendon in Essex would have been colonies. The predominant social philosophy at the time would have been one of social and gender separation and eugenics, the gradual elimination of the weakest.

The early 1970s saw a number of public enquiries into the standard of care in many of these large hospitals, including South Ockendon in Essex and Ely in Cardiff (Gilbert, 2009). Largely as a result of these public enquiries, better services for those with a learning disability were designed, those with a learning disability were seen as consumers of care and in the 1990s there arose an increase in disability rights and equality. There was also the growth of small family-sized community homes, reflecting an increase in community integration.

The 21st century sees the continued growth in social inclusion, human and civil rights, citizenship and self-advocacy (Gilbert, 2009). 'Mental handicap' becomes 'learning disability'. The old hospitals closed and care was (and is) provided in much smaller community-based homes. Many of those with a learning disability were encouraged to live semi-independently in their own homes with multi-agency support. These changes have been supported by anti-discrimination legislation including the *Disability Discrimination Act* in 1995, the *Valuing People* White Paper in 2001 and the Equality Act in 2010. All of these had an impact upon those with a learning disability and will be discussed further in *Chapter 4*.

2.4 **What it means to have a learning disability**

PAUSE FOR THOUGHT 2.4

Marcel has Down's syndrome. Is he 'learning disabled' or does he have a 'learning disability'? To put this question another way: is Marcel disabled or does he have a disability?

This question may not be either as simple or as rhetorical as it may at first seem. After all, in the previous section one can see how the use of language such as 'idiots', 'lunacy', 'mentally subnormal', 'mental handicap' and 'learning disability' changed over time and helped frame how those with a learning disability were viewed and treated.

A sign noticed in a church: 'INVALID TOILET'. Does this mean that this toilet is in-valid, not/non-valid? Or does it mean that those who use it are somehow in-valid, not valid? If it is the latter, what, then, is a valid person? Who decides and on what criteria?

In one way, we can never really understand and appreciate what it means to those like Marcel to have a learning disability, as such meanings are often value-laden, subjective and personal to every person who has a disability. After all, it is often claimed by those on the autism spectrum, for example, that if you meet one person with autism then you have met one person with autism! However, many are likely to experience discrimination, hate-motivated crime, infantilising attitudes, a lack of understanding and poor care on the part of some (but by no means all) care professionals. It could be suggested that one of the reasons for such experiences is the nature of the disability model that has been used in order to engage with those with a learning disability. There have been three main theoretical models that have sought to explain disability: the bio-medical model, the social model of disability (Hallawell, 2009) and the biopsychosocial model (Engel, 1977). The key characteristics of each are listed below:

2.4.1 Bio-medical model

- The person with a learning disability is seen, addressed and treated as a patient
- The role of the patient is to comply with medical, nursing and social 'treatment'
- The focus is on the disability: the individual is considered to be disabled due to his or her impairment
- The person is defined by his or her disability
- The language around disability is one of negative terms, of deviance, lacking normality
- The disability prevents the person from fully engaging within society
- The person with disability has to change in order to fit into society.

2.4.2 Social model

- Although originating in the mid-1970s, the social model came to prominence in the 1990s
- It has been described as being vaguely 'Marxist' in orientation
- It suggests that there is a difference between 'impairment' (such as sensory or physical impairment or learning disability) and 'disability'
- It looks beyond the individual impairment or disability to examine the social, political, educational and environmental causes of disability
- It is society that causes and imposes disability on the individual due to its ignorance, stereotyping and the erection of structural, physical, environmental and attitudinal barriers that prevent full engagement, inclusion and participation of the individual with a disability or impairment within society
- A positive disability identity and a pride in having a disability develops out of a greater control by those with a disability of both their own lives and the services that are provided for them

■ An aspect of this greater control by those with a disability is independent living supported with assistance when needed, rather than communal and dependent living.

2.4.3 The biopsychosocial model

Originating in 1977, George Engel's biopsychosocial model went on to become very influential and is the currently accepted model of care. According to this model, health and illness are determined by the interaction of three factors:

■ Biological (e.g. genetics, disease, physical trauma, brain damage, etc.)
■ Social (e.g. life traumas, early life experiences, family relationships, poverty, etc.)
■ Psychological (e.g. negative interpretation of events, emotions, beliefs, etc.)

There are a range of other models of disability in addition to the more commonly accepted medical, social and psychological models:

2.4.4 Expert or professional model

■ This model has provided a traditional response to disability issues and can be seen as an offshoot of the medical model.
■ Within its framework, professionals follow a process of identifying the impairment and its limitations (using the medical model), taking the necessary action to improve the condition of the disabled person.
■ This has tended to produce a system in which an authoritarian, overactive service provider prescribes and acts for a passive client.

(Disabled World, 2021)

2.4.5 Tragedy and/or charity model

■ Depicts disabled people as victims of circumstance who are deserving of pity.
■ This, along with the medical model, is the model most often used by non-disabled people to define and explain disability.

2.4.6 Moral model

■ People are morally responsible for their own disability. For example, the disability may be seen as a result of bad actions of parents (smoking, alcohol or drug use during pregnancy by the mother, for example) if congenital.

2.4.7 Empowering model

■ Allows for the person with a disability and their family to decide the course of their treatment and what services they wish to benefit from.
■ This, in turn, turns the professional into a service provider whose role is to offer guidance and carry out the client's decisions.
■ In other words, this model 'empowers' the individual to pursue their own goals.

2.4.8 Economic model

■ Defines disability by a person's inability to participate in work
■ It also assesses the degree to which impairment affects an individual's productivity and the economic consequences for the individual, employer and the state

■ Such consequences include loss of earnings for the individual and payment for assistance by them, lower profit margins for the employer and state welfare payments

■ This model is directly related to the charity / tragedy model.

2.4.9 Market model

■ A minority rights and consumerist model of disability that recognises people with disabilities and their stakeholders as representing a large group of consumers, employees and voters.

■ This model looks to personal identity to define disability and empowers people to chart their own destiny in everyday life, with a particular focus on economic empowerment.

Many of these models of disability are likely to influence and feed into a wide range of health and social care delivery as well as discussions around social welfare and welfare benefits, with politicians and political parties taking different standpoints.

2.5 Conclusion

This chapter has presented a number of different meanings and perspectives of learning disability. As a result, you should have acquired a basic understanding of what learning disability is and some of the statistics associated with having a learning disability. The meaning and understanding of learning disability is very much multi-dimensional in nature; differences in meaning and hence understanding arise from light being shone on learning disability from a variety of different angles, from a variety of different perspectives. Again, the meaning and understanding of learning disability have changed over time and will continue to do so. This is normal!

CHAPTER SUMMARY

Key points to take away from *Chapter 2*:
- ☑ There is no single definition of 'learning disability'.
- ☑ The ways in which learning disability and its attendant health issues can affect a person are manifold.
- ☑ It is important to be aware of and understand a basic history of learning disability before the current situation can be understood and to prevent historical mistakes being repeated in the future.
- ☑ There are different theoretical models of care, the main ones being 'social' and 'bio-medical'.

Questions

Question 2.1	Why is it important to have a clear understanding of the meaning of learning disability?

Question 2.2	What are likely to be possible impacts on people with a learning disability if you are not aware of and do not understand their political, social and legislative history?

Question 2.3	Which model of disability best fits your own thinking and resultant nursing practice and that of your colleagues with regard to those with a learning disability, and why?

Question 2.4	How could you use the various models of disability to improve the nursing care that you give to those with a learning disability and their families?

REFERENCES

Barber, C. (2011) Understanding learning disabilities: an introduction. *British Journal of Healthcare Assistants*, 05:04, 169–70.

British Dyslexia Association (undated) *About dyslexia*. Available at: www.bdadyslexia.org.uk/dyslexia/about-dyslexia/what-is-dyslexia (accessed 30 December 2021).

Department of Health (2001) *Valuing People: a new strategy for learning disability for the 21st century*. HMSO. Available at: https://assets.publishing.service.gov.uk/government/uploads/system/uploads/attachment_data/file/250877/5086.pdf (accessed 30 December 2021).

Disabled World (2021) *Definitions of the models of disability*. Available at: www.disabled-world.com/definitions/disability-models.php (accessed 30 December 2021).

Engel, G.L. (1977) The need for a new medical model: a challenge for biomedicine. *Science*, 196(4286): 129–36.

Garvey, F. and Vincent, J. (2006) 'The bio-physical aspects of learning disabilities'. In Peate, I. and Fearns, D. (eds) *Caring for People with Learning Disabilities*. John Wiley & Sons.

Gilbert, T. (2009) 'From the workhouse to citizenship: four ages of learning disability'. In Jukes, M. (ed.) *Learning Disability Nursing Practice*. Quay Books.

Hallawell, B. (2009) 'Challenges for the curriculum in learning disability nursing'. In Jukes, M. (ed.) *Learning Disability Nursing Practice*. Quay Books.

Heuser, S. (2012) 'The human condition as seen from the cross: Luther and disability'. In Brock, B. and Swinton, J. (eds) *Disability in the Christian Tradition*. Wm. B. Eerdmans Publishing.

Mencap (undated) *What is a learning disability?* Available at: www.mencap.org.uk/learning-disability-explained/what-learning-disability (accessed 30 December 2021).

New Scientist (2009) A rational alternative to testing IQ (editorial). *New Scientist*. Available at: www.newscientist.com/article/mg20427322-400-a-rational-alternative-to-testing-iq/ (accessed 30 December 2021).

NHS (2018) *Overview: learning disabilities*. Available at: www.nhs.uk/conditions/learning-disabilities (accessed 30 December 2021).

Public Health England (2016) *Learning Disabilities Observatory: People with learning disabilities in England 2015*. Available at: www.gov.uk/government/publications/people-with-learning-disabilities-in-england-2015 (accessed 30 December 2021).

Romero, M. (2012) 'Aquinas on the corporis infirmitas: broken flesh and the grammar of grace'. In Brock, B. and Swinton, J. (eds) *Disability in the Christian Tradition*. Wm. B. Eerdmans Publishing.

World Health Organization (2010) *International Statistical Classification of Diseases and Related Health Problems (ICD-10)*. WHO.

Chapter 3

Nursing support for those with profound and multiple learning disabilities

AIMS AND LEARNING OUTCOMES

The aims of this chapter are to:

3.1 Explore what profound and multiple learning disability (PMLD) is

3.2 Highlight the areas of care that a person who has a PMLD is likely to express, experience and need meeting using Roper, Logan and Tierney's 'twelve activities of daily living' as a model.

By the end of this chapter, you will be able to:

3.3 Understand and discuss what PMLD is

3.4 Discuss with a colleague or group of colleagues how the 'twelve activities of daily living' model of care could be used with a person who has a PMLD

3.5 Apply these twelve activities of daily living by appropriately incorporating them into care plans when working with a person who has a PMLD, tweaking these twelve activities when needed to meet specific care needs.

3.1 Introduction

Chapter 2 highlighted a number of possible definitions and meanings of learning disability and suggested that the various meanings of learning disability are intimately bound up with the use of language, and that as language changes, so does our understanding of those with a learning disability. It was suggested also that learning disability is a spectrum of conditions ranging from 'borderline' to 'profound'.

This chapter will highlight the needs and care of Thomas, a 65-year-old gentleman with a profound and multiple learning disability (PMLD) who has recently had a heart attack. Although Thomas lives in a small care home, he was admitted to an intensive care ward and then transferred to a medical ward of his local general hospital. Whilst set against the backdrop of a busy medical ward, the contents of this chapter will have value for those working in other hospital-based clinical areas, community services and care and nursing homes, as those with a PMLD are also likely to access these services or clinical areas.

This chapter will provide a simple 'definition' of what PMLD is, briefly explain one model of holistic care and then explore how this model of care can be applied to those with a PMLD.

SCENARIO 3.1

Thomas is a 65-year-old gentleman who lives in a social care home and has a profound and multiple learning disability (PMLD) with additional needs in the following areas:
- Severe mobility problems; is unable to sit without assistance and mobilise without the use of a wheelchair
- Pre-verbal communication skills; needs assistance to communicate
- Inability to digest food and drinks due to dysphagia; requires assistance to eat and drink
- Arthritis
- Epilepsy
- Pain management
- Taking and monitoring medication and their side-effects
- Doubly incontinent
- Personal hygiene; needs help with washing and bathing.

Thomas has suffered a heart attack and has been admitted to the ward on which Sally, the senior staff nurse introduced in *Chapter 1*, works.

3.2 What is PMLD?

It is notoriously difficult to estimate with any precision the number of those with a PMLD in the UK. However, it is very roughly estimated that there are between 40 000 and 45 000 people who have a PMLD (PMLD Link, 2017).

Those with a PMLD, as well as having a profound learning disability (as indicated by an IQ of less than 40), are likely to have more than one significant disability which could include:
- neurological issues such as epilepsy
- physical disabilities such as cerebral palsy which will impact on the person's mobility
- significant communication, eating and drinking problems
- respiratory and cardiovascular problems, sensory impairments, mental health issues, 'classic autism'
- increased health problems that could be associated with any or all of the above.

People with a PMLD are thus very likely to need significant additional support in order to maintain an optimum level of health and to engage within society.

3.3 Twelve activities of daily living

Student nurses in all four pre-registration fields of practice are taught the vital importance of assessing the holistic needs of the patient or service user and then planning, implementing and evaluating a therapeutic and supportive care plan that meets these assessed needs. This process of assessing, planning, implementing and evaluating care intervention is known as the 'nursing process'. This nursing process utilises the work of three nursing theorists (Nancy Roper, Winifred Logan and Alison Tierney); this work is the 'twelve activities of daily living' (ADLs) (Roper, Logan and Tierney, 2000).

The twelve activities of daily living are:
- maintaining a safe environment
- communication
- breathing
- eating and drinking
- elimination
- washing and dressing
- controlling temperature
- mobilisation
- working and playing
- expressing sexuality
- sleeping
- death and dying.

These twelve activities of daily living often serve as a useful structure for patient or service user assessment and resultant care planning, usually within a hospital setting. As Thomas is likely to experience and express a need for a high level of support in virtually all areas of his life, this model of assessment and support will be utilised. However, mental health, neurological issues such as epilepsy, emotional care and spiritual care appear to be missing from this particular care model, so it is important to take these additional elements into account to ensure that the healthcare assessment and resultant care and support package are truly holistic.

3.3.1 The role of the nurse

Within this current context, the first role of the nurse is to reassure Thomas, who is likely to be anxious if not downright scared. Do not forget that Thomas is likely to be in pain and confused, as he is in an unfamiliar environment and among people that he does not know. All of these are likely to increase his anxiety levels.

The second priority for the registered nurse and possibly the nursing associate is to assess holistically Thomas's needs with a 'strengths and needs' model, using the framework suggested by the twelve activities of daily living. Parts of this assessment may be relatively straightforward to complete and record, whilst other aspects may be less so. Do not forget to involve Thomas, any care staff from his care home and his family (if appropriate) in this assessment as much as possible, as not only will much useful information be gathered this way but it is also good practice. After all, if you were a hospital patient, would you like your own care needs assessed and a care package planned for you without your involvement? Ideally, any care assessment and resultant care planning should be done on a multidisciplinary basis, and this must include the views of the patient. Check and use any 'hospital passbook' that may accompany Thomas, as this is likely to contain much useful information about Thomas's likes, dislikes and needs as well as how his needs are usually met. Any resultant care plans must likewise be holistic and incorporate Thomas's views, likes and dislikes.

3.3.2 Maintaining a safe environment

Thomas, along with everyone else, needs a safe environment in which to live. Maintaining a safe environment for Thomas is likely to include assessing many of the following:

- Does Thomas have a history of falls, epilepsy or ear infections that may affect his balance?
- Does Thomas have any known allergies that could impact upon the care and support that he receives whilst in the hospital?
- Does Thomas require any specific manual handling equipment and if so, is this equipment such as hoists and slings regularly serviced and maintained?
- Does Thomas require mobility assistance, such as a wheelchair?
- Does Thomas require assistance to maintain healthy skin and prevent the occurrence of skin tissue breakdown such as pressure sores and ulcers?
- Does Thomas require any specific 'feeding equipment' such as percutaneous endoscopic gastrostomy (PEG) equipment in order to maintain optimum nutrition and if so, is this feeding equipment regularly cleaned, serviced and maintained?
- Are nursing and other care staff adequately and appropriately trained to use any equipment that Thomas needs to maintain optimum health?
- Is Thomas's immediate environment free from unacceptable and inappropriate risks, such as clutter?

Nurse's role
- Carry out an assessment that could include some, many or all of the questions suggested above, on the environmental factors that impact upon Thomas's care
- Action any issues highlighted in this assessment
- Do so in collaboration with other members of the multidisciplinary team (MDT) including Thomas, his carers and his family (if appropriate).

3.3.3 Communication

Thomas has very little verbal communication skill and is limited to grunts, groans, cries and the occasional scream. Thomas communicates through facial expression, body language, basic Makaton and the occasional 'verbalisation'. Makaton is a sign language that was derived from British Sign Language and is used with and by people with a learning disability and, more recently, those with Alzheimer's dementia. Makaton is a language programme using signs and symbols to help people to communicate; it is designed to support spoken language and the signs and symbols are used with speech, in spoken word order (Makaton Charity, undated).

Thomas has a variety of communication problems and needs (Griffiths and Doyle, 2009). These include making himself understood, understanding others, and having to rely on others to interpret what he is trying to say.

It is imperative that, at least initially, Sally take her cue from the care home staff that have accompanied Thomas. Once Sally gets to know Thomas, she should build upon her observations of Thomas and the way that he communicates with his care home staff and initiate conversations with him. Never forget, communication is a basic human need, and the ability and freedom to communicate a basic human right.

Nurse's role
- Carry out a baseline assessment on Thomas's communication abilities and needs, based in part on observations
- Learn simple and basic Makaton signs (a speech and language therapist should be able to assist here)
- Adapt one's own communication forms so as to engage directly with Thomas rather than with Thomas's care home staff.

3.3.4 Breathing

As Thomas has had a heart attack, the quality and quantity of his respiration may be affected. This must be monitored, appropriate support offered, and outcomes recorded. Thomas's posture may also impact negatively upon his ability to breathe properly. Therefore, the input of a physiotherapist or occupational therapist may be required to ensure that Thomas is sitting or lying correctly and that his posture is not impeding his ability to breathe. The following useful resources provide further information on postural care and learning disabilities:

- Mencap (undated) *PMLD – Postural care. Available at:* www.mencap.org.uk/advice-and-support/profound-and-multiple-learning-disabilities-pmld/pmld-postural-care (accessed 30 December 2021).
- Public Health England (2018) *Postural care and people with learning disabilities: guidance. Available at:* www.gov.uk/government/publications/postural-care-services-making-reasonable-adjustments/postural-care-and-people-with-learning-disabilities (accessed 30 December 2021).

Nurse's role
- Assess and document the quantity and quality of Thomas's respiration
- Check oxygen saturation levels
- Reposition Thomas to maximise his ability to breathe unaided
- Liaise with physiotherapists and doctors to maximise Thomas's ability to breathe unaided
- Consider the option of oxygen therapy
- Assist with the devising and implementation of care plans that will help Thomas to breathe unaided
- Evaluate and document the outcomes of such care plans.

3.3.5 Eating and drinking

Thomas, like many other people with a PMLD, experiences dysphagia (difficulty in swallowing) and requires all of his food and drink to be the consistency of a 'thickish' paste. This involves having his meals puréed and his drinks thickened with a proprietary thickener such as Thick & Easy. For dietary advice, food consistency levels and use of terminology regarding diet and dysphagia, contact the local speech and language therapist and dietitian. The International Dysphagia Dietary Standardisation Initiative (IDDSI) has developed a framework that provides a common terminology to describe food textures and drink thickness (IDDSI, 2019).

It must never be forgotten, however, that the consumption of food and drink is not just a mechanical or biophysical process as it involves the physical, emotional and psychological sensations of smell, taste and touch, as well as incorporating sociocultural and memory elements. Having a PMLD must not preclude Thomas from engaging in eating and drinking as pleasurable social and cultural activities and experiences.

In order to maintain optimum nutritional levels and balance and for the optimum administration of medicines, the possibility of percutaneous endoscopic gastrostomy (PEG) is being considered. For Thomas this is an endoscopic medical procedure in which a tube is passed into a patient's stomach through the abdominal wall and through which nutrition / food, drinks and medicines will be passed (PEG feeding).

ACTIVITY 3.1

Ask a colleague to either assist you to eat a small and simple puréed meal such as a small plate of fish and chips or cheese and egg salad, or to feed you a puréed meal. You are not allowed to verbally communicate throughout this activity, but you can use signs and facial expressions. After the meal, record your thoughts and feelings, focusing on what it felt like to be fed and the approach, attitude and communication of your colleague.

Nurse's role
- Be aware of and understand the social and cultural aspects of eating and drinking
- Carry out an assessment of Thomas's likes, dislikes, nutritional needs and eating / drinking abilities and challenges, recording the assessment outcomes
- Make meal times as relaxed, calm and pleasant as possible
- Liaise with other care professionals including speech and language therapists, nutritionists, physiotherapists and occupational therapists to make eating and drinking easier and more comfortable for Thomas.

3.3.6 Elimination

PAUSE FOR THOUGHT 3.1

"…Good morning Thomas. Oh, you've messed your bed again."

I know, it's not my fault and anyway I have had to lie in it for the last hour.

(paraphrased from Griffiths and Doyle, 2009, p. 285)

- How do you think Thomas feels at being told that he has messed his bed again?
- How do you think Thomas feels about not being checked, cleaned and changed before now?

Those with PMLD, like Thomas, are very likely to experience both urinary and faecal incontinence (Griffiths and Doyle, 2009). As a senior staff nurse, Sally is likely to participate in the assessment of Thomas's continence levels and abilities and the impact that such incontinence has on the quality of Thomas's life.

Nurse's role
- Monitor the side-effects of any medicines that Thomas may be taking; all medicines have side-effects and some of these may affect his levels of urinary and faecal continence
- Be aware of the range and types of continence aids that are available; disability product retailers / suppliers such as NRS Healthcare and trade fairs such as Naidex may be useful here
- Ensure that any continence aids that Thomas normally uses at his care home continue to be used whilst on the hospital ward; this ensures continuity of care
- Ensure that any continence aids such as pads are used appropriately and correctly, are fit for purpose, fit Thomas comfortably, do not leak, are changed regularly and are not visible underneath his clothing
- Ensure that Thomas's personal hygiene needs are met
- If appropriate and possible, encourage Thomas to use 'ordinary' toilet facilities, bearing in mind that his mobility is decreased
- Ensure that Thomas's abilities and needs are reviewed regularly
- If changes to the type of continence aids are suggested / recommended as a result of reviews, ensure that this is communicated properly to Thomas's care home staff.

3.3.7 Washing and dressing

Thomas requires assistance with all aspects of personal hygiene, oral hygiene and dressing. This involves the choosing of cleaning and personal and oral hygiene products, the choosing and purchasing of clothing and choosing which items of clothing to wear on any given day. Thomas, being doubly incontinent, is likely to require extra assistance to maintain optimum personal hygiene. Such assistance must be offered gently, sensitively and with the utmost care and attention to detail, including privacy.

Nurse's role

- Carry out a full assessment of Thomas's washing and dressing needs, recording the outcomes of this assessment
- Be aware of and understand the social and cultural significance of personal hygiene and forms of clothing
- Encourage Thomas to be as independent as possible, offering assistance as and when needed
- Be aware of 'adaptive clothing'; disability product retailers / suppliers such as NRS Healthcare and disability trade fairs such as Naidex may be useful here
- Liaise with other care professionals such as occupational therapists.

3.3.8 Controlling temperature

As Thomas is unable to tell you whether he is hot, cold or feels 'just right', let alone to control his own temperature, Sally will need to be aware of any subtle changes in his behaviour (whether, for example, he appears more agitated or aggressive or less engaged and communicative than usual), in facial expression and body language. Sally will also need to report and record these subtle changes as they form most of Thomas's communication repertoire, and then act upon them.

Nurse's role

- Offer to decrease or increase the amount of clothing that Thomas wears
- Offer hot or cold drinks
- Increase or decrease the amount of bed covering (blankets) that Thomas has
- Increase or decrease the 'ambient' room or environment temperature through the use of small fans or portable heaters, if appropriate and safe
- Monitor, report and record the effects, if any, on Thomas's behaviour and how he communicates.

3.3.9 Mobilisation

Thomas has profound mobility problems and is unable to walk. However, he is able to weight bear for very short periods of time and to stretch out his arms. These abilities must be encouraged and may be useful in helping Thomas to get dressed and undressed. The advice and support of Thomas's care home staff, the physiotherapist and the occupational therapist are likely to be essential to maximise Thomas's mobility capacity. Although unable to walk, Thomas does own and use a purpose-built wheelchair and this wheelchair must be maintained and utilised whilst he is on Sally's ward.

Nurse's role
- Assess and record Thomas's mobility skills and challenges
- Contribute to care planning
- Respect and promote Thomas's mobility and dexterity independence as far as possible
- Liaise with other care professionals such as physiotherapists and occupational therapists; the physiotherapist, for example, would also be able to advise on a range of simple physical exercises that could prevent muscle and joint pain and keep his joints and limbs working and mobile
- Contribute to the implementation of agreed care plans.

3.3.10 Working and playing

It is unlikely that those with a PMLD are able to work in the same way and on the same basis that Sally is able to. It will be unrealistic for those with a PMLD to obtain and hold down a paid job in a shop, an office, a factory or on a hospital ward as an HCA or nurse or go to the local pub at the end of a nursing shift. However, without being patronising or condescending, those with a PMLD are capable of engaging in a number of 'work-related' activities around the house and at any daycare facilities that they may attend. Thomas, for example, enjoys assisting with the housework and the preparation of meals and cooking where he lives. This he does through holding the vacuum cleaner's hose pipe and pushing it across the floor, holding a duster and wiping the table tops and mixing food (such as a cake mixture) in a bowl or helping to make sandwiches. Thomas may need assistance to understand why he cannot engage in these activities whilst on Sally's hospital ward.

Thomas does enjoy going out shopping and for a coffee and accessing the countryside near where he lives. It may be appropriate for Thomas to be assisted to visit the hospital café or restaurant and shop whilst he is in hospital.

Nurse's role
- Understand the importance of meaningful activity, work and leisure in people's lives
- Understand the impact on a person's physical and mental wellbeing if such meaningful activity, work and leisure opportunities are unavailable
- Explain to Thomas why he cannot engage in his daily activities and routines – the use of alternative forms of communication such as line drawings and photos may be helpful
- Arrange visits to the hospital coffee shop, restaurant and shop (most hospitals will have these facilities; Heartlands hospital in Birmingham, for example, has a restaurant that sells Starbucks coffee and an M&S food shop). Ensure that care home staff, friends or family that visit are made aware of these facilities and allow them to take Thomas off the ward.
- If Thomas does not receive any visitors, it may be necessary for the ward staff to take Thomas off the ward for a while, enabling him to access these facilities
- Record the impact, positive and negative, on Thomas after he has accessed these facilities and amend the care plan accordingly.

3.3.11 Expressing sexuality

Of all the twelve ADLs, this is likely to be one of the two most contentious and difficult for nursing and other care staff to work with. Yet human sexuality is a crucial aspect of the human identity and what it means to be human. Thomas, despite having a PMLD, has the same sexual drives and needs as anyone else. However, expressing sexuality involves more than just the physical act of sex, as it also encompasses such diverse elements as clothing styles, use of cosmetics, hair styles, use of language, social and employment activities and even the music one listens to.

Nurse's role
- Understand how all these elements impact upon the person who is Thomas
- Be aware of and understand how Thomas expresses his sexuality
- Safeguard and promote his individual choices
- Ensure that his right to privacy is recognised, safeguarded and promoted.

PAUSE FOR THOUGHT 3.2

Consider what it would feel like if your own sexuality and sexual expression was either controlled or denied by other people.

3.3.12 Sleeping

Thomas experiences occasional problems in sleeping at night due, in part, to his tendency to sleep during the day because of under-stimulation and boredom, and his need to be turned regularly at night in order to prevent tissue breakdown. A number of issues need to be addressed here:

Nurse's role
- Thomas's sleep pattern needs to be monitored and recorded; this must involve an assessment of both quantity and quality of sleep as well as Thomas's anxiety levels, comfort (noise levels, whether he is too hot or cold, pain levels and the suitability of the bed and mattress) and the actual timing of his sleep patterns
- Thomas needs to be kept fully engaged in social activities during the day
- Disruption to Thomas's night-time sleep pattern must be kept to a minimum and recorded when it does occur
- Thomas's medication may need to be reviewed, as insomnia may feature as a side-effect of some pre-existing medication and the introduction of 'night-time sedation' may need to be considered (although this is likely to be a last resort measure).

3.3.13 Death and dying

As with sexuality, death and dying is one of the two most contentious ADLs. Whilst Thomas shares this ultimate destiny with all of humanity and, indeed, with all living things, this is not to say that Thomas will die or is likely to, whilst in Sally's care. Nonetheless, the possibility of Thomas's death must be acknowledged and accepted and possibly factored into his care.

Nurse's role

- Reassure Thomas and explain to him what is happening in ways that he can understand
- Reassure and explain to Thomas's family what is happening to him
- Ascertain what a 'good living', a 'good dying', a 'good death' and a 'good after death' look like for Thomas
- Ascertain whether Thomas has membership of any religion or has attended any form of religious service – if Thomas has and with his permission, contact his faith community leader of choice (priest, vicar, minister, rabbi, imam, etc.) and request a hospital visit
- *DO NOT* offer to pray for Thomas or impose your own religious views or identity but DO participate in any form of spirituality or religious services if appropriate and required
- Liaise and work with other members of the hospital care team, including the hospital chaplaincy team if appropriate, Thomas's family and Thomas's care home staff, in relation to end of life care (whether these needs are perceived or actual)
- Work mindfully around Thomas (this could also be good practice when working with any other patient or service user) – for more on mindfulness see the work of Jon Kabat-Zinn.

ACTIVITY 3.2

Arrange to meet and discuss end of life issues with a member of your local hospital chaplaincy team and specialist end of life and bereavement nurses, focusing on the holistic, person-centred care and support that Thomas and his family may need during the dying, death and bereavement stages.

3.4 Conclusion

As can be seen from the above, PMLD affects Thomas in virtually every aspect of his life. It is likely that, at some point in Sally's career as a staff nurse or nurse manager, she will come into contact and work with patients like Thomas, so the aim of this chapter is to provide a small number of suggestions as to how Sally can work with and meet the needs of those with a PMLD within a hospital setting. However, be warned: the use of the 'twelve activities of daily living' and other similar assessment and care planning models is not to be carried out as a sterile 'tick box' activity, nor to be written in stone. Those with a PMLD deserve and have a right to better than that. Such models are to be seen and used as guidance for appropriate care assessment and planning only.

CHAPTER SUMMARY

Key points to take away from *Chapter 3*:
- ☑ It is estimated that there are between 40 000 and 45 000 people in the UK who have a PMLD.
- ☑ PMLD can be defined as having an IQ level of below 40 and with a wide range of additional physical, neurological and sensory disabilities.
- ☑ One of the models of care that may be useful in meeting the holistic care needs of those with a PMLD is the twelve activities of daily living devised by Roper, Logan and Tierney.
- ☑ Caution must be exercised in not turning this care model into a 'tick box' method of caring.

Questions

Question 3.1   How would you describe to a colleague what profound and multiple learning disability is?

Question 3.2   How could you use the twelve activities of daily living (ADLs) to provide nursing care to someone like Thomas?

Question 3.3   Are there any aspects of a person's life (such as mental health, spirituality and religion, for example) that are missing from the '12 ADLs'? If so, how would you fill any areas of care that you think may be missing from the '12 ADLs'?

Question 3.4   How would you prevent the '12 ADLs' from becoming a 'tick box' exercise?

REFERENCES

Griffiths, C. and Doyle, C. (2009) 'Nursing people with profound and multiple learning disabilities'. In Jukes, M. (ed.) *Learning Disability Nursing Practice*. Quay Books.

IDDSI (2019) *Complete Framework*. Available at: https://iddsi.org/IDDSI/media/images/Complete_IDDSI_Framework_Final_31July2019.pdf (accessed 30 December 2021).

Makaton Charity (undated) *About Makaton*. Available at: www.makaton.org/aboutMakaton (accessed 30 December 2021).

Mencap (undated) *PMLD – Postural care*. Available at: www.mencap.org.uk/advice-and-support/profound-and-multiple-learning-disabilities-pmld/pmld-postural-care (accessed 30 December 2021).

PMLD Link (2017) *Supporting people with profound and multiple learning disabilities*. Available at: www.pmldlink.org.uk/wp-content/uploads/2017/11/Standards-PMLD-h-web.pdf (accessed 30 December 2021).

Public Health England (2018) *Postural care and people with learning disabilities: guidance*. Available at: www.gov.uk/government/publications/postural-care-services-making-reasonable-adjustments/postural-care-and-people-with-learning-disabilities (accessed 30 December 2021).

Roper, N., Logan, W.W. and Tierney, A.J. (2000) *The Roper–Logan–Tierney Model of Nursing: based on activities of living.* Elsevier Health Sciences.

RESOURCES

Mencap: Profound and Multiple Learning Disabilities: www.mencap.org.uk/advice-and-support/profound-and-multiple-learning-disabilities-pmld (accessed 30 December 2021).

PMLD Link: www.pmldlink.org.uk (accessed 30 December 2021).

Chapter 4

Learning disability legislation and reports

AIMS AND LEARNING OUTCOMES

The aims of this chapter are to highlight:

- The differences between the various forms of legislation and associated documents

- The various laws, White Papers and reports that have an impact specific to those with a learning disability

- A number of issues within these documents that have a specific impact upon nurses and nursing practice.

By the end of this chapter, you will be able to:

- Describe and discuss the differences between a Parliamentary Bill, a Parliamentary Act, a Green Paper, a White Paper and an independent report

- Describe and discuss the various pieces of legislation and associated documents that have a specific impact upon those with a learning disability

- Discuss how these various documents may impact upon your own nursing practice.

PAUSE FOR THOUGHT 4.1

Those who are not aware of and do not understand their history are condemned to repeat its mistakes: discuss!

4.1 Introduction

The area of health and social care law, Green Papers, White Papers and reports is both fascinating and complex. It can certainly be confusing and frustrating! Yet, not to have a working knowledge and understanding of these relevant Government documents that impact upon the lives of those with a learning disability could, and probably will, have serious consequences on the quality and forms of services that people with a learning disability receive. Understanding these government documents and policies will help you to both comply with the law and provide high-quality care to people with a learning disability.

It must be stated here that those who have a learning disability are subject to the same laws, both civil and criminal, as everyone else in society; having a learning disability does not exclude the person from the consequences, rights, **protection** and responsibilities of the law and their conduct under the law, and neither should it! However, there are a number of laws that have a specific impact upon those with a learning disability and these will serve as the basis for this chapter.

This chapter will highlight the contents and the impact of the wide variety of Parliamentary Bills, Parliamentary Acts, White Papers and reports that impact upon the lives of those with a learning disability over the past 40 years.

4.2 Differences between Bills, Acts, White Papers, Green Papers and reports

It seems almost like every day that this, that or the other Bill, Act, report or whatever is released and highlighted in the daily newspapers, on radio and TV. There is no way that we, as members of society, can ignore such media attention and debate into what may often seem to be rather dry, obscure, obtuse and even apparently irrelevant issues. And neither should we. As nurses, as healthcare professionals, we live and work in a legislation-rich environment and that is the way it has always been, always will be and indeed must be!

There are a number of differences between a Parliamentary Bill, a Parliamentary Act, a Green Paper, a White Paper and an independently commissioned report (see *Table 4.1*). You can read more about how laws are made on the UK Parliament website at: www.parliament.uk/about/how/laws/.

A **Parliamentary Bill** is an intended piece of legislation which originates from either the House of Lords or the House of Commons. Some Bills start life as part of the annual Queen's Speech to Parliament and then become part of the Government's legislative programme, whilst others are presented and sponsored by a backbench MP (any backbench MP can present and sponsor a Parliamentary Bill) or a member of the House of Lords. An example of the former could include the Care Bill 2013 and an example of the latter could include the Autism Bill 2009 which was sponsored by Cheryl Gillan (MP). A Bill does not have any legal authority in itself and cannot be treated and implemented as a law, as many Parliamentary Bills do not pass all the required Parliamentary stages and become law. The sole exception to this is the annual Finance Bill (the Budget) which often contains measures (such as increases in tobacco, alcohol and petrol/diesel prices) that are immediately implemented on the day of the budget.

Table 4.1 *Key features of the main forms of UK legislative documents*

Document	Key features
Parliamentary Bill	<ul><li>An intended piece of legislation</li><li>Originates from either the House of Lords or the House of Commons</li><li>Some Bills start life as part of the annual Queen's Speech to Parliament and then become part of the Government's legislative programme</li><li>Others are presented and sponsored by a backbench MP (any backbench MP can present and sponsor a Parliamentary Bill) or a member of the House of Lords</li></ul>
Parliamentary Act	A Parliamentary Bill that has successfully completed its parliamentary journey, been presented to and signed by the sovereign (the Queen or King), acting in their capacity as Head of State
Green Paper	A discussion or consultation document that is issued by political parties around specific issues such as mental health, transport or the environment
White Paper	A policy document that is often published by the Government
Independent report	<ul><li>A report into specific events or issues</li><li>Often written or commissioned by organisations, such as Mencap, that are outside of formal government structures</li></ul>

A **Parliamentary Act** is a Parliamentary Bill that has successfully completed its parliamentary journey, been presented to and signed by the sovereign (the Queen or King), acting in their capacity as Head of State. Then, and only then, does it have any legal power and can be implemented. Some Parliamentary Acts serve to prohibit certain actions or behaviour of individual citizens or organisations, whilst others permit certain actions or behaviour. An example of the former could include the law which banned smoking in public places like pubs, cafés and restaurants. An example of the latter could include the Abortion Act 1967, which permitted legal abortions under certain conditions.

So, how exactly does a Bill become law?

Taking the 2009 Autism Bill as an example, its parliamentary journey included first and second readings, committee stage, report stage and third reading in the House of Commons. This process was then repeated in the House of Lords. The Autism Bill returned to the House of Commons where any amendments proposed by the Lords were debated and either accepted, amended or discarded. Once consensus had been reached by both Houses of Parliament, the Bill was presented to the Queen for signing. Once signed by the Queen (as Head of State), the Autism Bill became the Autism Act 2009.

A **Green Paper** is a discussion or consultation document that is issued by political parties around specific issues such as mental health, transport or the environment, whereas a **White Paper** (such as *Valuing People* (DH, 2001)) is a policy document that is often published by the Government. One of the purposes of a White Paper is to present service delivery guidelines which, although not mandatory, would be very good practice if they were to be implemented.

An **independent report** is a report into specific events or issues and is often written or commissioned by organisations, such as Mencap, that are outside of formal government structures. Examples of such reports could include the Report of the Mid Staffordshire NHS Foundation Trust Public Inquiry, also known as the Francis Report (TSO, 2013), Mencap's *Death by Indifference* (2007, 2012) and the report into the abuse of people with a learning disability who were residents at Winterbourne View hospital in 2011. These independent reports often serve as a catalyst both for changes in how services are organised and delivered, and for the amendment or generation of new legislation.

4.3 Key documents relating to learning disabilities

In this section we will look briefly at a number of important documents that have an impact on the care of people with learning disabilities.

4.3.1 Better Services for the Mentally Handicapped (1971)

- This White Paper came about partly as a result of a number of highly critical reports into the standard, type and quality of care that those with a learning disability received at a number of mental handicap (learning disability) hospitals in England and Wales.
- It recommended halving the number of hospital places for those with a learning disability.
- Long-stay hospital settings for people with learning disabilities should gradually be closed and replaced with residential and 'day care' support in the community.
- Personal assessment of service user needs and greater involvement of the families of those with a learning disability were highlighted (Concannon, 2005).

4.3.2 Jay Report (1979)

- The Jay Report was set up under the chairmanship of Mrs Peggy Jay.
- The Report called for a review of learning disability nurse training in line with the philosophy of independent living (an emancipatory philosophy and practice which empowers disabled people and enables them to exert influence, choice and control in every aspect of their life (Hasler, 2003)).
- The Report was highly critical of large institutional forms of service provision which did not allow for community engagement.
- Those with a mental handicap / learning disability had the right to live in an ordinary house in an ordinary street and to use and benefit from ordinary community resources.

- The framework of services should be one that both respects the person with a learning disability who uses the service and meets the person's needs.
- The Report recommended that mentally handicapped adults (adults with a learning disability) should have residential provision in or near the social and geographical communities in which they spent their childhood or early adulthood (Concannon, 2005).

4.3.3 Mental Health Act 1983

- This was the first piece of mental health law since 1959.
- *Part 1 / Section 1*: sets out the legal definition of learning disability (mental and severe mental impairment) as being an "arrested or incomplete development of mind which includes a significant or severe impairment of intelligence and social functioning".
- *Part 2 / Sections 2–5*: allows for compulsory or voluntary admission to hospital, for either assessment or treatment of a serious mental health issue. *Section 5* allows doctors and mental health / learning disability nurses to prevent those with serious mental health issues, and who are at risk of harming themselves or others, from leaving a hospital.
- *Parts 3–5*: deal with patients concerned in criminal proceedings or who are under sentence, consent to treatment (more on this in *Chapter 6*) and mental health tribunals.

4.3.4 NHS and Community Care Act 1990

- This Act introduced an 'internal market' into the supply of health and social care within England, Scotland and Wales.
- The State (local authorities) became considered more an 'enabler' / broker than a direct health and social care provider for those with a learning disability and their families.
- Local authorities were tasked with taking the lead in enabling social care assessment and provision for those with a learning disability.
- The Act restructured the NHS into NHS Trusts and included the establishment of 'fund-holding' GP practices.
- The Act highlighted the rights of those with a learning disability to be active participating members of their local communities, living and working within that community (Kelly, 2006).
- The Act provided assistance to allow those with a learning disability to remain in their own home, should they wish (Fearns, 2006).

4.3.5 Disability Discrimination Act 1995

- This Act made discrimination on the grounds of disability (including learning disability) an offence.
- It defined what disability meant.
- It placed a duty on employers not to discriminate against employees or employment applicants on grounds of disability (McIver, 2006).

- The employer had a duty to make adjustments to the application and selection process in terms of recruitment processes and to the work premises and environment (including any equipment used by the employee).
- *Part 3* of the Act placed a duty on service providers in a wide range of areas to provide appropriate and reasonable disability access to their premises and equality of treatment once on the premises.
- *Part 4* made it an offence to discriminate against or disadvantage pupils/students (including those with a learning disability) on the grounds of any disability that they may have.
- *Part 5* gave the Government powers to make regulations relating to the design and accessibility of public transport.
- *Part 6* created the National Disability Council.

4.3.6 *Valuing People* (2001)

- This was first White Paper for 30 years that deals specifically with those with a learning disability.
- It comprised eleven key objectives, most of which have a direct impact upon nursing care:
  1. Maximising life opportunities for children with a learning disability through ensuring optimum access to and use of educational, health and social care services whilst maintaining the child at home
  2. Transition into adult life through ensuring continuity of educational, health and social care and support for the young person and their family
  3. Enabling more control and choice over their own lives through a person-centred approach to planning
  4. Increasing the help and support that the 'informal' caregivers receive from local authorities
  5. Enabling people with learning disabilities to access a high-quality health service designed around their individual needs
  6. Enabling those with a learning disability and their families to have a greater choice of where and how to live
  7. Enabling people with learning disabilities to lead full and meaningful lives in their communities and to develop a range of friendships, activities and relationships
  8. Enabling more people with learning disabilities to make a valued contribution to the world of work through participating in all forms of paid employment
  9. Ensuring that all care agencies commission and provide high-quality, evidence-based, cost-effective and continuously improving services
  10. Ensuring that social and health care staff working with people with learning disabilities are appropriately skilled, trained and qualified
  11. To promote holistic services for people with learning disabilities through effective partnership working between all relevant local agencies in the commissioning and delivery of services.

4.3.7 Mental Capacity Act 2005

- This Act promotes and safeguards the right to make decisions and to accept and refuse any healthcare, social care, nursing and medical interventions, if the person has the capacity to do so.
- Those with a disability, including those with a learning disability, cannot be denied the right to make decisions for themselves purely on the grounds of their disability.
- It safeguards those who, for whatever reason, do not have mental capacity.
- It allows for advance decisions to refuse treatment and for the establishment of a 'lasting power of attorney' (someone who can decide and act on behalf of another person).
- For a more in-depth discussion on the Mental Capacity Act 2005 and its implications and applications for nurses working with those with a learning disability, see *Chapter 6* of this book.

4.3.8 Mental Health Act 2007

- This Act amended and reformed the Mental Health Act 1983.
- It defines mental disorder as *"any disorder or disability of the mind"*.
- The definition is wide enough to include not only mental illness, but also learning disability, autism and personality disorders.
- Learning disability in Section 1(4) is *"a state of arrested or incomplete development of the mind which includes significant impairment of intelligence and social functioning"*.
- Because this definition would place learning disability within the definition of mental disorder, Section 1(2A) provides that learning disability will not constitute mental disorder unless it is *"associated with abnormally aggressive or seriously irresponsible conduct"* on the part of the patient, such as requiring treatment in a hospital for mental health conditions. This proviso is important because neither Section 3 (dependence on alcohol or drugs) nor Section 7 (medical treatment) of the Act will apply to a learning disabled person unless the Section 1(2A) qualification is met. Thus, a person with a learning disability will come under the purview of the 2007 Act only if they express abnormally aggressive (violent) or seriously irresponsible behaviour which will impact upon mental capacity.
- It is worth noting that the MHA 2007 is being updated to become more empowering and person-centred/needs-led, the Deprivation of Liberty Safeguards are being replaced by Liberty Protection Safeguards and interact with the Mental Capacity Act and Mental Health Act again to improve culture and working practices around capacity.

4.3.9 *Death by Indifference*

- Mencap published *Death by Indifference* following the deaths of six people with a learning disability in NHS care (Mencap, 2007).
- It exposed the unequal healthcare and institutional discrimination that people with a learning disability often experienced within the NHS.

- *Death by Indifference* played an important role in influencing the Department of Health to commission the confidential enquiry into premature deaths of people with a learning disability.
- The Report called for learning disability liaison nurses to be established in all acute general hospitals to act as advisors to ward staff.

4.3.10 Autism Act 2009

- This is the first disability-specific piece of law in the UK.
- The Act makes provision for and offers guidance about meeting the needs of adults with autistic spectrum conditions on the part of local authorities and the NHS through the 'Autism Strategy'.
- Specific areas highlighted by this Act include diagnosing, identification and assessment of adults who are on the autism spectrum.
- The Act recommends holistic planning in relation to the provision of relevant services to people with autistic spectrum conditions as they move from being children to adults, and the training of staff who provide relevant services to adults with such conditions.

4.3.11 Equality Act 2010

- The Equality Act supersedes the Disability Discrimination Act of 1995.
- It seeks to reduce socioeconomic inequalities and eliminate discrimination, and prohibit victimisation on a wide range of grounds (protected characteristics) including: age, disability, gender, sexual orientation, marital status, ethnic background and religion and belief.
- Reasonable adjustments will be made to service provision and premises access.
- For those who believe that they are discriminated against, remedies through the civil courts and employment tribunals are laid out.

ACTIVITY 4.1

- Discuss with a colleague what you consider to be the meaning of 'reasonable adjustment' within your work setting.
- Apply this meaning to a person with a learning disability with whom you work.

4.3.12 *Death by Indifference: 74 deaths and counting*

- This is a five-year review and progress report that is based on the 2007 Mencap report *Death by Indifference*.
- Following on from the 2007 report, a further 68 deaths of those with a learning disability in general acute hospitals have come to light.
- Issues that were highlighted in both the original 2007 and the current progress reports include: lack of care for patients who have a learning disability, poor communication, failure to recognise pain, failure to monitor patients' health conditions, and diagnoses and treatment of healthcare conditions were delayed.
- Do Not Resuscitate orders were made inappropriately, purely on the grounds of a patient having a learning disability.

- Provisions and intentions of the Mental Capacity Act 2005 were routinely ignored. Doctors were rarely formally sanctioned or reprimanded by the General Medical Council (GMC) for these deaths.
- Mencap made a number of recommendations including training for all healthcare professionals in relation to those with a learning disability, awareness of avoidable deaths and the identification and tracking of patients who have a learning disability whilst accessing healthcare services.
- Mencap suggested that family and other carers should be involved as a matter of course as partners in the provision of treatment and care.
- All Trust Boards should demonstrate in routine public reports that they have effective systems in place to deliver effective, 'reasonably adjusted' health services for those people who happen to have a learning disability.
  (Mencap, 2012)

4.3.13 CIPOLD 2013

- The Confidential Inquiry into premature deaths of people with learning disabilities (CIPOLD) resulted from the Mencap *Death by Indifference* report.
- It explored the reasons behind the untimely deaths of those with a learning disability, along with associated health issues and disparities.
- The CIPOLD study has shown the continuing need to identify people with learning disabilities in healthcare settings, and to record, implement and audit the provision of 'reasonable adjustments' to avoid their serious disadvantage.
- Proactive use of Annual Health Checks to develop and implement Health Action Plans, planning for the future and adapting care as needs change rather than in a crisis, and the identification of effective advocates to help people with learning disabilities to access healthcare services are all effective, low-cost measures to address this issue. Professionals must recognise their responsibilities to provide the same level of care to people with learning disabilities as to others, and not to make rapid assumptions about quality of life or the appropriateness of medical or social care interventions.

4.3.14 Children and Families Act 2014

- This Act made provision about children, families and people with special educational needs or disabilities; it made provision about the right to request flexible working; and for connected purposes.
  - Part 1: Adoption
  - Part 2: Family justice (covers welfare of the chid and care plans)
  - Part 3: Children and young people in England with special educational needs or disabilities (this includes education, health and care plans and provision). This is likely to be the most important part of this Act when working with children and young adults with a learning disability and their families.

4.3.15 Care Act 2014

- This was an Act to make provision to reform the law relating to care and support for adults (with health and disability issues) and the law relating to support for (informal) carers
    - to make provision about safeguarding adults from abuse or neglect;
    - to make provision about care standards;
    - to establish and make provision about Health Education England;
    - to establish and make provision about the Health Research Authority;
    - to make provision about integrating care and support with health services; and for connected purposes.
- It covers assessing and meeting of needs by local authorities along with charges for social care provision.

4.3.16 LeDeR reviews

- LeDeR (formerly known as the Learning from Deaths Review programme) is a service improvement programme which aims to improve care, reduce health inequalities and prevent premature mortality of people with a learning disability and autistic people (NHS England and NHS Improvement, 2021).
- LeDeR reviews are about looking at the life of a person with a learning disability and/or who is autistic who died, and finding out about the health and social care services which that person received throughout their life.
- It is not a mortality review because its purpose is not to find out why that person died, nor is it an investigation into their death.
- It is about assessing the type and quality of received care so that improvements to health and social care services can be made.

4.4 Suggestions for further research

- Obtain and read through the various reports, particularly the 2007 and 2012 Mencap reports. The reports, both in full and the 'executive summary', are readily available online. Briefly summarise their main points. Ask yourself whether the apparent discrimination that is implicit within these reports could occur where you work and what your response should be. Your response should be guided by local circumstances and protocols and the experiences of those with a learning disability and their families.
- Find, download and read the Mental Capacity Act 2005, Equality Act 2010, Care Act 2014 and the Children and Families Act 2014. Briefly summarise the main points within each of these Acts that are likely to affect your practice as a nurse.
- Speak to those with a learning disability (the local learning disability liaison nurse should have contact details of local Mencap and Down's Syndrome Association groups, along with local self-advocacy groups that may be useful). Summarise the Care Act 2014, Children and Families Act 2014 and the Equality Act 2010 in an easy to understand format and present these to those with a learning disability. Ask those with a learning disability how they would like you to promote their legal, civil and human rights under these laws.

- 'Disability discrimination should be consigned to the dustbin of history'. Is disability discrimination still an issue and will it continue to be an issue for the foreseeable future where you live and work, despite the existence of the above reports, White Papers and laws? If it is, should this be the case and what can you do to challenge it?
- Take one of the parliamentary Acts, White Papers or independent reports highlighted in this chapter. How would you set about using the chosen document within a presentation on healthcare law that you have been asked to give to your nursing and medical colleagues?

4.5 **Conclusion**

This chapter has attempted to highlight a number of laws, White Papers and reports that have had a direct impact upon both the lives of those with a learning disability and on healthcare / service provision for this patient group over the past four decades. Understanding these government documents and policies is likely to prove rather challenging but may help you to comply with the law and to provide high-quality care to people with a learning disability.

CHAPTER SUMMARY

Key points to take away from *Chapter 4*:
- ☑ There have been a number of pieces of legislation (Acts of Parliament / laws) and reports over the past 40 years that have had a direct impact upon the lives of those with a learning disability.
- ☑ Some of these have been as a direct result of a shift in thinking and attitudes towards those with a learning disability.
- ☑ Others have been as a direct result of poor-quality nursing, medical and social care. The ultimate aim of these laws and reports is to improve the lives of those with a learning disability.
- ☑ The reading, understanding and implementation of these laws and reports are likely to prove challenging but worthwhile.

Questions

Question 4.1   What are the differences between a law, a Bill, a White Paper, a Green Paper and an independent report?

Question 4.2   How does a parliamentary Bill become a parliamentary Act?

Question 4.3   How would you encourage your MP to present a Bill to Parliament on an issue that you feel very strongly about in connection to those with a learning disability?

Question 4.4   Take one of the parliamentary Acts, White Papers or independent reports highlighted in this chapter. How would you set about using the chosen document within a teaching session on healthcare law that you have been asked to present to your colleagues?

REFERENCES

CIPOLD (2013) *Confidential Inquiry into premature deaths of people with learning disabilities (CIPOLD)*. Norah Fry Research Centre. Available at: https://www.bristol.ac.uk/media-library/sites/cipold/migrated/documents/fullfinalreport.pdf (accessed 2 January 2022).

Concannon, L. (2005) *Planning for Life: involving adults with learning disabilities in service planning*. Routledge.

Department of Health (2001) *Valuing People: a new strategy for people with learning disability for the 21st century*. Available at: www.gov.uk/government/publications/valuing-people-a-new-strategy-for-learning-disability-for-the-21st-century (accessed 2 January 2022).

Fearns, D. (2006) 'Protecting "vulnerable" adults with learning disabilities'. In Peate, I. and Fearns, D. *Caring for People with Learning Disabilities*. John Wiley & Sons.

Hasler, F. (2003) *Philosophy of independent living*. Available at: www.independentliving.org/docs6/hasler2003.html (accessed 2 January 2022).

Kelly, J. (2006) 'Working with adults with learning disabilities'. In Peate, I. and Fearns, D. *Caring for People with Learning Disabilities*. John Wiley & Sons.

McIver, M. (2006) 'Legislation and learning disabilities'. In Peate, I. and Fearns, D. *Caring for People with Learning Disabilities*. John Wiley & Sons.

Mencap (2007) *Death by Indifference.* Available at: www.mencap.org.uk/sites/default/files/2016-06/DBIreport.pdf (accessed 2 January 2022).

Mencap (2012) *Death by Indifference: 74 deaths and counting (a progress report 5 years on).* Available at: www.mencap.org.uk/sites/default/files/2016-08/Death%20by%20Indifference%20-%2074%20deaths%20and%20counting.pdf (accessed 2 January 2022).

NHS England and NHS Improvement (2021) *Learning from lives and deaths – People with a learning disability and autistic people (LeDeR) policy 2021*. Available at: www.england.nhs.uk/wp-content/uploads/2021/03/B0428-LeDeR-policy-2021.pdf (accessed 2 January 2022).

The Stationery Office (2013) *Report of the Mid Staffordshire NHS Foundation Trust Public Inquiry*. Executive summary available at: https://assets.publishing.service.gov.uk/government/uploads/system/uploads/attachment_data/file/279124/0947.pdf (accessed 2 January 2022).

FURTHER READING / RESOURCES

Legislation

Autism Act 2009: www.legislation.gov.uk/ukpga/2009/15/contents (accessed 2 January 2022).

Care Act 2014: www.legislation.gov.uk/ukpga/2014/23/contents (accessed 2 January 2022).

Children and Families Act 2014: www.legislation.gov.uk/ukpga/2014/6/contents/enacted (accessed 2 January 2022).

Disability Discrimination Act 1995: www.legislation.gov.uk/ukpga/1995/50/contents (accessed 2 January 2022).

Equality Act 2010: www.legislation.gov.uk/ukpga/2010/15/contents (accessed 2 January 2022).

Mental Capacity Act 2005: www.legislation.gov.uk/ukpga/2005/9/contents (accessed 2 January 2022).

Mental Health Act 1983: www.legislation.gov.uk/ukpga/1983/20/contents (accessed 2 January 2022).

National Health Service and Community Care Act 1990: www.legislation.gov.uk/ukpga/1990/19/contents (accessed 2 January 2022).

UK Parliament *How are laws made?* Available at: www.parliament.uk/about/how/laws/ (accessed 2 January 2022).

White Papers / reports

Department of Health and Social Security / Welsh Office (1971) *Better Services for the Mentally Handicapped.* HMSO.

Jay, P. (1979) *The Report of the Committee of Enquiry into Mental Handicap Nursing and Care.* Department of Health.

LeDeR (2017) Available at: https://leder.nhs.uk/about (accessed 2 January 2022).

Chapter 5
Medical care and support for those with a learning disability

---

AIMS AND LEARNING OUTCOMES

The aims of this chapter are to:

- Highlight the support needs of those with a learning disability who access general healthcare facilities

- Highlight some of the barriers and issues that many people with a learning disability face whilst accessing healthcare services

- Set out a broad range of measures and interventions that could be put into place when working with this service user group within a 'general healthcare' setting such as a GP practice, a hospital ward or an outpatient department.

By the end of this chapter, you will be able to reflect on, describe, discuss and, where relevant, apply and/or meet:

- The care needs of a patient with a learning disability

- A number of barriers faced by those with a learning disability when they access healthcare facilities

- A number of measures and interventions that could be utilised to overcome these barriers.

5.1 Introduction

Most nurses and other health and social care professionals are likely at some point in their work to meet and provide general healthcare support and services to those with a learning disability within a number of healthcare settings. Such settings could include an Accident and Emergency (A&E) department, a general practice or health centre, an outpatient department, a surgical or medical ward or a dental practice. This chapter will focus on a number of practical issues that those with a learning disability may encounter when accessing such generalist healthcare services and settings.

ACTIVITY 5.1

Discuss with a colleague how you as a nurse or healthcare professional would provide high-quality support to those with a learning disability within the environment where you work.

In order to do this, you may like to consider the following:
- Person-centred holistic assessments
- Person-centred care planning
- MDT working
- Knowing who to ask for advice and knowing the right questions to ask
- Acknowledging the limitations of your knowledge and skills when working with this patient group.

5.2 Healthcare needs of those with a learning disability

SCENARIO 5.1

Ziva, a woman in her 30s who has high-functioning autism / Asperger's syndrome (HFA/AS) and is a university lecturer, and who also has a son with classic autism, is to be admitted to a gynaecological ward where Sally works as an occasional bank nurse, for a planned minor operation to remove uterine polyps by hysteroscopy.

SCENARIO 5.2

Marcel, a young man in his 30s with Down's syndrome who lives at home with his parents and is Ziva's brother, attends a pre-arranged 1 pm appointment at a local hospital's 'lumps and bumps' clinic (where, again, Sally works as an occasional bank nurse) for a large and painful cyst on his finger, having been referred to this clinic by his GP.

As Public Health England (PHE, 2018) states:

> *"Individuals regardless of their age, gender or label should receive care that is based on their unique needs, that is appropriate in its design and effective in its delivery."*

PHE points out that people with learning disabilities have more healthcare needs than the general population and that about 50% of people with a learning disability will have at least one significant health problem. In addition, those with a learning disability will experience the same health conditions and have the same health needs as everyone else. Many of these are relatively routine and commonplace, such as:
- flu
- respiratory, skin and other infections
- diabetes
- weight management
- musculoskeletal issues including gout

- minor injuries
- pain management
- smoking cessation
- health education
- health screening
- vaccinations
- ongoing community-based support for issues such as heart problems, dementia, strokes and mental health
- dementia care
- family planning, gynaecology and reproduction, contraception and pregnancy.

These should be dealt with by the GP or practice nurse in the same way as anyone else but with additional support as and when needed. However, there is evidence that suggests there is poor provision and uptake of relatively common screening and health management opportunities such as cervical screening in women with a learning disability; such poor provision and uptake stems from stigma regarding learning disability and health care and may result in further stigma (Byrnes *et al.,* 2019).

Some forms of minor injury such as those incurred during sports activities, for example, and other health conditions may need the input of appropriate 'out of hours' services, 'walk-in' minor injury units or A&E departments. But, again, this is normal and many people without an additional learning disability will use these services at some point in their lives.

Other health conditions may require a more specialist medical or nursing input including:
- diagnosis and care of cancers
- diagnosis and care of dementia
- complex issues around gynaecology
- strokes and heart attacks
- renal issues
- endocrine and neurological disorders.

Again, this is normal and is part and parcel of being human. Indeed, Barber (2001) made this clear in his paper on the professional development of nurses with regard to those on the autism spectrum. Although Barber's focus was on those with an autism spectrum condition twenty years ago, his point is applicable to those who have a learning disability today.

However, many of those with a learning disability will experience specific health conditions often associated with their specific form of learning disability or syndrome. For example, respiratory, circulatory and cardiac problems are often associated with people who have Down's syndrome (see the checklist given in Down's Syndrome Association (2021) and RCGP (undated) as indicators of the forms of health issues that those with a learning disability are likely to experience). Again, prevalence of epilepsy is often higher in those with a learning disability than elsewhere in society (Epilepsy Action, 2018).

In previous decades, most relatively minor healthcare interventions for those with a learning disability were carried out within the old mental handicap hospitals. By 'relatively minor' is meant the type of healthcare issues one would usually see the GP, community nurse, optician or dentist about. Indeed, such hospitals tended to be very self-contained and provided more or less everything that the person with a learning disability needed. However, with the closure of these large and often isolated hospitals during the 1980s and 1990s, the provision of healthcare services was transferred to mainstream acute and community healthcare providers.

5.3 Roles of the nurse

There are a number of specific practical suggestions that could be useful to nurses, HCAs, student nurses and other health and social care professionals when working within a generalist healthcare setting. Such settings are likely to include a GP practice or community health centre, an A&E or out of hours unit, an outpatient unit or a surgical or medical ward. Some of the following practical suggestions may be more useful than others, whilst some may be easier to implement and may be cheaper to act upon than others. However, quality must never be sacrificed in order to keep down costs. Do not forget that the framework suggested by the twelve activities of daily living in order to provide high-quality holistic care, highlighted in *Chapter 3*, could be useful here.

PAUSE FOR THOUGHT 5.1

What do you consider to be the steps required to ensure that Ziva and Marcel are admitted 'hassle free' to the ward or department where Sally works?

As a first step, the nurse or other health and care professional, when working with a person with a learning disability, must be aware of the possibility for 'diagnostic overshadowing' which is defined as "once a diagnosis is made of a major condition… a tendency to attribute all other problems to that diagnosis, thereby leaving other co-existing conditions undiagnosed" (Neurotrauma Law Nexus, undated). In other words, health conditions may be seen as a consequence of having a learning disability rather than as health conditions in their own right and treated accordingly (Blair, 2017). The nurse needs to see beyond the diagnosis and 'label' of learning disability to both the health condition and the person with that health condition. It must never be forgotten that the person with a health condition is a person first and has the right to be engaged with as such.

5.3.1 Access the support of the learning disability liaison nurse

In order to provide better support for both Marcel and Ziva during their stay at the hospital, a learning disability liaison nurse (LDLN) would be invaluable. An LDLN is a specialist learning disability trained nurse who supports people with a learning disability while they are in hospital to make sure they get the care they need.

Where there is an LDLN, it's important that they meet the patient as soon as possible after they arrive at the hospital. This is so that the LDLN can find out everything they need to know about the patient's learning disability and health condition and the help they will need while in hospital. It may be possible to arrange a meeting before the hospital stay.

The learning disability liaison nurse can assist with:
- coordination of care – at points of attendance, admission and discharge
- education within clinical areas and contributing to programmes of education
- support and advice for acute care staff in relation to personalised care and service delivery
- collaboration between the agencies involved in service delivery to ensure effective seamless care by undertaking home visits
- development and enhancement of standards of care for all patients with a learning disability attending the acute hospital
- promotion of effective communication with those involved in the patient's care – whether they are community- or hospital-based
- support of a relative or a family member with a learning disability who is affected by the patient's illness / hospital stay
- promoting safety and minimising risk
- provision of accessible information about treatments
- promotion of positive experiences and outcomes (NHS Lothian, 2020).

ACTIVITY 5.2

Arrange to meet your local learning disability liaison nurse and discuss any concerns that you may have about meeting the nursing needs of any previous, current or potential future patients / service users with a learning disability who may be in your care.

5.3.2 Assess, assess and assess

This may sound obvious, but it is imperative that every service user or patient who has a learning disability must be treated as an individual. It may therefore not be appropriate to approach, assess or treat:
- a young child with a learning disability in exactly the same way as you would a teenager or an adult with a learning disability, or
- a person with severe or profound learning disability in the same way as a person with a mild or moderate learning disability.

Each of these people will have differing information, care and support needs. Therefore, not only must the patient assessment be absolutely thorough, but it must be holistic, person-centred, appropriate to the individual and fit for purpose. It may be necessary to use a set of assessments that have been devised specifically to meet the communication needs of those with a learning disability, or to adapt or amend existing assessment tools that may not address those needs directly. For example, it may be necessary to substitute words and numerical scales with simple line drawings or pictures. One such example could be the Wong–Baker FACES® Pain Rating Scale (*Figure 5.1*) where service users are asked to choose one of six faces that best depicts the pain they are experiencing.

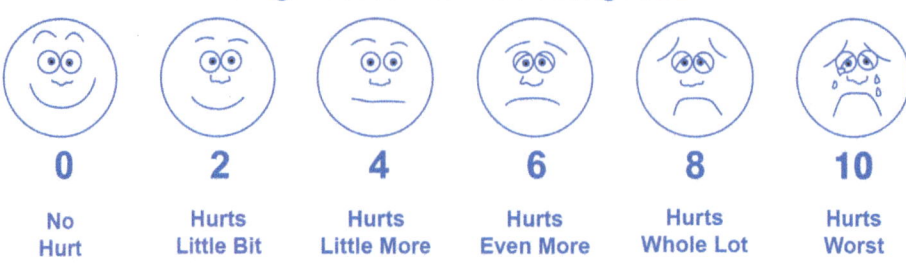

Figure 5.1 *Wong–Baker FACES® pain rating scale.*

ACTIVITY 5.3

Discuss with a colleague how you could adapt existing nursing assessment tools to make these useable for those with a moderate and a severe learning disability.

5.3.3 Accessible information

It is vital for the service user or patient with a learning disability to have information that is simple, easy to understand, timely, accurate, and in a format that the patient can use. Although Ziva works as a university lecturer, the manner in which she processes information, particularly when stressed, may require such information to be presented in ways other than written or verbal. As the information levels and needs will vary from person to person and from condition to condition and even from day to day, the type and level of information that is offered will likewise have to vary, as will the ways in which this information is presented. Such communication issues will be highlighted during assessments.

It is important, here, to be imaginative and creative in how appropriate information is offered, particularly within tight financial and time constraints. However, what must be borne in mind when providing information to people with a learning disability is that without appropriate information, the patient's or service user's ability to give informed consent to treatment will be threatened and may even not exist. This could have potentially profound practical, legal and ethical consequences for both the patient and the nursing and medical staff.

ACTIVITY 5.4

Produce a simple and 'easy read' leaflet that explains to a potential patient with a learning disability the services offered in the clinical environment where you work. Try to obtain the funding necessary to print such a leaflet.

5.3.4 Communication

Communication is the central key, the linchpin to everything that the nurse does with the patient or service user and is essential in order to gain consent to any intervention or care. It must be borne in mind that communication is not a one-way process (e.g. from nurse to patient) but is an active multiway process involving a minimum of two people but likely to involve many more. However, the person with a profound learning disability, such as Thomas from *Chapter 4*, may be totally non-verbal or may communicate through facial expressions and other forms of body language, through pre-verbal 'grunts' or through sign languages such as Makaton (a simpler form of British Sign Language). Therefore, it is vital for Sally to take the time and really observe, to really get to know the patient so that she can pick up on the various hidden nuances in their behaviour, facial expressions and body language in order to ascertain what it is they are communicating.

In order to communicate, particularly with those who may be 'less-abled', imagination may be needed in presenting or acquiring information effectively. Similarly, imaginative forms of communication may be required when engaging in social communication with a person with a learning disability such as chatting about the weather, the football results or even just saying 'hello'.

ACTIVITY 5.5

Reflect and note down how and why you could change the way you communicate with a person with a moderate and severe learning disability.

5.3.5 Pre-admittance visits

If it is feasible, arranging pre-admittance visits for patients who have a learning disability may be very useful in order to familiarise that person with the routines, procedures, sights, sounds, smells and people within a hospital ward, outpatient department or dental surgery. Cumella and Martin (2000) cite examples of hospitals arranging such visits, recording video footage of 'life on a hospital ward' for those with a learning disability or preparing very simple pre-admittance information sheets and leaflets using a combination of actual photos, pictures and line drawings. NICE (2019) suggests that people growing older with a learning disability should meet hospital staff before any planned hospital admission, to agree arrangements that make the stay easier for them.

However, such pre-admittance visits can be resource-intensive and prohibitive in terms of money and time and in an environment that is increasingly budget-conscious, it may be difficult to justify such resources for what could be a relatively small number of patients. Having said that, do contact and talk to the learning disability liaison nurse for advice on how to produce accessible pre-admittance information. Also, by using relatively scarce resources in an imaginative and creative manner, it may be possible to produce simple and cheap information and videos for those with a learning disability. Finally, the Mencap website (www.mencap.org.uk) may provide useful suggestions regarding pre-admittance visits and information.

ACTIVITY 5.6

How would you arrange a pre-admittance visit by a person with a learning disability onto the ward or department on which you work? Write down your thoughts and discuss them with a colleague.

5.3.6 Timing of appointments

SCENARIO 5.2– CONTINUED

Marcel, a young man in his 30s with Down's syndrome, attended a pre-arranged 1 pm appointment at a local hospital's 'lumps and bumps' clinic for a large and painful cyst on his finger, having been referred to this clinic by his GP. When Marcel arrived at this clinic, there were about a dozen other people waiting to be seen. A notice appeared on the clinic wall advising the patients that there was a 50-minute delay, which stretched to 55 and then 60 minutes. Marcel did not understand the delay or the reason for it and rapidly became agitated and anxious. Marcel started to pace up and down the waiting area, becoming more verbally and then physically agitated and aggressive, scratching and biting himself on his arms. The clinic staff asked the hospital security to escort Marcel out of the clinic and the hospital, saying that his behaviour was disruptive and was scaring other patients. Consequently, because Marcel was not seen by the clinic, his cyst was not diagnosed at this appointment as being pre-cancerous, which it actually was.

PAUSE FOR THOUGHT 5.2

How would you support Marcel in this particular situation?

Many of those with a learning disability, particularly those who are also on the autism spectrum, will have set and rigid daily routines which, if disrupted, may result in a 'behaviour meltdown'. Again, many of those with a learning disability will experience anxiety and stress and perhaps extreme anxiety if exposed to unfamiliar environments, smells and sounds and unexplained delays. Thus, it is important to keep disruption and resultant anxiety to an absolute minimum. One way to achieve this is to schedule medical appointments for fairly quiet times, either very early appointments or the last appointments of the day, so that there are fewer people around and noise levels are lower, which will lead to lower levels of sensory stimulation and arousal. If Marcel or Ziva need to visit the GP practice, health centre or outpatient department for any reason it may also be helpful to book a 'double appointment' in order to allow time for information to be given to the patient and for the patient to be able to ask questions regarding their health and treatment.

It would be very helpful if Marcel and Ziva could have any GP appointments with the same GP at each appointment. This would allow the GP and the patient to get to know each other and the patient would not feel that they have to repeat themselves to different doctors whom they see. It would certainly be helpful not to have a 'general appointment time' but, instead, to have specific appointment times. A nine o'clock appointment must mean 09.00 and not 09.30 or 10.00. This is less likely to heighten anxiety levels with a resultant 'behavioural meltdown' such as was experienced and expressed by Marcel. If appointments are delayed significantly for any reason, and in the real world this may very likely be the case, ongoing explanations for the delay and reassurance using language and terms that the patient with a learning disability is likely to understand, would be useful. As with Marcel, it may be helpful to lead the patient into a quiet room or area or to allow the patient to 'jump the queue'.

ACTIVITY 5.7

Reflect on the possible impact on and consequences for a person with a learning disability who is having to wait over an hour for their outpatient appointment, and then note down three things that you can do to ensure that people are seen at the time given on their appointment letter.

5.3.7 Hospital passports

PAUSE FOR THOUGHT 5.3

What, if anything, is wrong about the following question: *"Does he take sugar?"*

Northway *et al.* (2017) reviewed 60 hospital passports in use in the UK and found that they could enhance patient safety and person-centred care, but that they varied considerably in format and in the information contained. Some standardisation is required, but typically such documents (which may also be referred to as 'personal passbooks', 'communication passports', etc.) would include the following information:

- A photograph of the person
- Information about key contacts and health needs
- The patient's likes and dislikes
- How they communicate
- Any dietary needs and food allergies
- Mobility issues
- Personal care issues
- Personal faith community contacts if needed
- Any medication that is being taken.

If nurses and HCAs are familiar with and read such passbooks, the need to ask whether the patient takes sugar in his tea or coffee becomes largely redundant.

However, as a way of starting a conversation with a patient who has a learning disability, it may be useful to ask the patient if he or she has sugar in their coffee or tea. The point here is that the question should become "Do *you* take sugar?" rather than "Does *he* take sugar?" and could be used as social politeness in the same way as with any other person. Marcel would very much prefer it if the health professionals caring for him were to talk to him, not at or about him! However, those with a learning disability may not be able to verbally communicate, thus it is imperative to read their passbook and communicate with them in ways that they can understand and participate in.

Each hospital is likely to have its own version of this type of passbook but the format of using simple language and pictures to present information is likely be very similar. This passbook will be completed by the person with a learning disability or by someone who knows this person well. If such a passbook does not exist where Sally works, it may be worth contacting the learning disability liaison nurse for advice on how to design and produce one.

ACTIVITY 5.8

Obtain a hospital passport from your local learning disability liaison nurse. Having read it, note any ways that the passport can be amended in line with the aims and objectives of your work environment.

5.3.8 Support during admittance

We are now going to consider support during admittance in the context of our two scenario patients.

SCENARIO 5.1 – CONTINUED: ZIVA

It may be helpful for Ziva to receive a text message the day before her appointment to remind her. Ziva, who was accompanied to the hospital by her husband, could be met at the hospital entrance by a 'buddy'. Such a 'buddy' could be arranged by the hospital's LDLN and may well be a volunteer. The role of the 'buddy' will be to explain to Ziva where her ward is and to take her there, to explain hospital and ward procedures and layout and to be a 'friendly face' in what can often be seen as a hostile and frightening environment. Once on the ward, a full medical history and assessment that is relevant to the procedure must be taken. Ziva must be fully involved in the assessment, being treated as a person and not as a medical condition. As part of this assessment, Ziva's mobility and self-care abilities will be considered.

As Ziva is articulate and is able to communicate verbally, a passbook is not likely to be needed. However, due to her Asperger's syndrome Ziva might ask for information to be offered initially using simple rather than complex language and jargon. She should be offered the opportunity to ask questions, which must be answered honestly. This could take place in a side room as this would be more likely to afford Ziva quietness and may be less stressful for her.

SCENARIO 5.1 – CONTINUED: MARCEL

Marcel was fully able to communicate with the hospital staff at the outpatients clinic that he attended. However, the clinic staff failed to communicate effectively with him and this caused Marcel a lot of anxiety and resulted in 'inappropriate behaviour' on his part, which in turn resulted in him being unable to attend his initial appointment. However, the hospital-based LDLN, who ideally should have been involved at the outset and even prior to Marcel's appointment, was able to intervene at the request of Marcel's parents and Marcel was offered another appointment at the clinic. During this second appointment, Marcel was supported by the liaison nurse and his parents.

ACTIVITY 5.9

Write down how you could make reasonable adjustments during the process of admitting a person with a learning disability onto your ward. Does this look any different from how you would admit a person who does not have a learning disability onto your ward?

5.3.9 Support before the procedure

As the named nurse for Marcel and Ziva, Sally will discuss with them the various options for their respective conditions (it is more likely that the permanent rather than the bank staff would act as the named nurse). With Ziva, the option would be whether to have her polyps removed by hysteroscopy under either local or general anaesthetic. Sally will assess Ziva's ability to process and understand information and explain to her what this procedure actually entails in terms that she will be able to understand. Sally will give Ziva an information leaflet on the procedure and answer any questions that Ziva has.

Marcel will be offered support from the LDLN during his second appointment. The LDLN will work with Sally to ensure that Marcel is made aware of any delays in being seen and the reasons for these delays, and that Marcel is reassured.

ACTIVITY 5.10

Write down three ways that you could support a patient with a learning disability *prior to* undergoing a surgical procedure. Are these the same as when supporting a 'non-learning disabled' person undergoing the same procedure?

5.3.10 Support during the procedure

Ziva will be offered the choice between having the polyps removed under local or general anaesthetic. If, as is likely, Ziva opts for the former, she will be conscious throughout. Therefore, the procedure will be explained to her step by step, while her husband could be given the option of using the staff room and having a welcome cup of coffee while he waits for her to return to the ward.

Marcel will be supported by the LDLN throughout his second appointment at the 'lumps and bumps' clinic. It will be suggested to Marcel that because of the small risk of the cyst being cancerous, a biopsy could be advisable. The liaison nurse will explain to Marcel and his parents what this means and what it will involve.

ACTIVITY 5.11

Write down three ways that you could support a patient with a learning disability who is undergoing a surgical procedure. Are these the same as when supporting a 'non-learning disabled' person undergoing the same procedure?

5.3.11 Support after the procedure

After the polyps are removed, Ziva will be taken back to the side room on the gynaecology ward and be offered pain relief, verbal reassurance and careful monitoring. Any questions that Ziva may have about the polyps and the procedure will be answered by her named nurse.

After the excision of the cyst for biopsy, Marcel will be given pain relief, an explanation of what should happen next, reassurance and a follow-up appointment.

In some senses, the care that both Marcel and Ziva should expect will be no different from the care that any patient undergoing similar, or indeed any, procedures should expect. However, given that Marcel, certainly, and Ziva to a certain extent, are going to experience language barriers due to their disabilities, it is important to be aware of the need to adapt communication styles and forms in order to offer reassurance and to ensure that the right information is given in the right way to facilitate understanding and consent.

ACTIVITY 5.12

Write down three ways that you could support a patient with a learning disability who has just undergone a surgical procedure. Are these the same as when supporting a 'non-learning disabled' person who has undergone the same procedure?

5.3.12 Discharge

Given that discharge planning should commence when the patient is admitted onto the ward or department and should not be seen as an afterthought at the end of the stay, the key to a successful discharge for both Ziva and Marcel will be communication, team working and appropriate referrals. As the nurse allocated to Ziva, Sally is likely to be involved in drawing up her discharge plan. Ziva must be offered information about general gynaecology as well as condition-specific aftercare in a format that she can access and understand, taking into account any communication and information processing issues that may affect those with Asperger's. Ziva should be reminded of the importance of having someone at home to look after her for a day or two. Ziva will be referred back to her GP for general check-ups and the results of tests that were carried out on the removed polyps, as some polyps may be cancerous in nature.

Marcel's discharge plan will likewise be thorough. Marcel and his parents will be offered easy to read information about the aftercare of a person who has had a cyst biopsy. A follow-up appointment should be made during which the results of the cyst biopsy will be explained. As a result of the biopsy, a referral to a cancer specialist should be made.

ACTIVITY 5.13

Consider the consequences for the patient if the discharge care plan is left to the last minute. Could or does this happen where you work? What actions could you take to ensure that any discharge care plans are 'fit for purpose'?

5.3.13 Follow-up

Follow-up in Ziva's case could be a phone call from the hospital learning disability liaison nurse two or three weeks after discharge. This would be to find out how she is now and how any follow-up appointments with her GP went.

Marcel would also be contacted by the learning disability liaison nurse and might receive home visits from the dietitian, the physiotherapist and the community learning disability nurse who might have liaised with the cancer specialists at the hospital. The community learning disability nurse would ensure that Marcel is resting and looking after himself properly. They would also arrange for any further health checks to be made.

ACTIVITY 5.14

Devise a simple protocol which sets out appropriate and costed post-discharge follow-up that will include the input and roles of all stakeholders and care professionals. If you are in a position to do so, obtain senior management approval for the protocol and then implement it.

5.4 Professional development opportunities

According to Mencap there are continuing failures in care for people with a learning disability and several reports related to poor care, some of which have resulted in the deaths of those with a learning disability and/or autism. Since March 2007 when Mencap published *Death by Indifference*, further deaths have been reported to Mencap, deaths which families blame on hospital blunders, poorly trained staff and indifference (Mencap, 2018). Again, there have been several reports into the abuses carried out at Winterbourne View and Whorlton Hall involving people with a learning disability and/or autism (DH, 2012; NHS England, 2014; BBC, 2019).

There is thus a need for nurses at all levels to receive awareness raising and basic training in learning disability care as part of their ongoing professional development programmes. This need was highlighted as a result of a government consultation exercise during the first few months of 2019.

The consultation was initiated after the death of the teenager Oliver McGowan, following which his mother Paula launched a parliamentary petition asking for all doctors and nurses to receive mandatory training in learning disability and autism awareness (see www.olivermcgowan.org for more details of the campaign). She argued fiercely that autism must be included in such training. On 22 October 2018, her petition was debated on the floor of the House of Commons and gained cross-party support. As a direct consequence the UK government announced that all NHS and social care staff would receive The Oliver McGowan Mandatory Training in Learning Disability and Autism. The need for such training was reinforced through the subsequent report on the government's consultation on the mandatory training of health and social care professionals regarding learning disability and autism (Department of Health and Social Care, 2019).

There are core capability frameworks for supporting people with learning disabilities and/or autism (see *Chapter 1* and the *Resources* section), and the Oliver McGowan Mandatory Training in Learning Disability and Autism is being developed (HEE, 2021) in conjunction with partners including Mencap and the National Autistic Society (Mencap, 2021). Opportunities for professional development will become available, and you will be expected to attain the capabilities appropriate to your level of role and to undertake the mandatory training.

ACTIVITY 5.15

Contact either the local or regional Mencap office or the hospital-based LDLN for advice and suggestions as to how to access appropriate training / professional development that would cover the issues of what learning disability is and is not, its causes, as well as how to provide high-quality care to a patient who has a learning disability.

5.5 Conclusion

Those with a learning disability are as likely as anyone else to experience health issues and illnesses that require either the support of community-based healthcare such as GP practices or admittance to a general hospital. Nurses' knowledge about learning disability care is historically not as good as it should be and this has contributed to the needless deaths in general hospitals that resulted in the 2007 Mencap report *Death by Indifference*. However, those with a learning disability have a right to high-quality healthcare and medical and nursing care and there is much that the nurse, student nurse and HCA working within a 'generalist' healthcare setting could do to ensure that high-quality care is delivered.

CHAPTER SUMMARY

Key points to take away from *Chapter 5*:
- ☑ Those with a learning disability are as likely to experience health issues and illnesses as anyone else.
- ☑ Historically, nurses and HCAs working in general healthcare settings are not trained to work with those who have a learning disability.
- ☑ There are a number of ways that hospital and community-based nurses could improve the quality of the nursing support experienced by those with a learning disability whilst accessing healthcare facilities.
- ☑ These include carrying out holistic assessments, providing appropriate information, pre-admission visits, timing of appointments, patient-held information 'passbooks' and communication.

Questions

Question 5.1 What are the healthcare needs of those with a learning disability?

Question 5.2 How would you assess the holistic care needs of a patient with a learning disability that is in your care?

Question 5.3 List ten barriers to accessing healthcare that are often faced by those with a learning disability. For each of these barriers, how would you challenge these barriers in your daily work?

Question 5.4 For each of the barriers that you have listed in your answer to *Question 5.3*, how would you assist a person with a learning disability to challenge and overcome them?

REFERENCES

Barber, C. (2001) The training needs of registered nurses engaged in work with people with an autistic spectrum disorder. *Good Autism Practice*, **2(2)**: 86–96.

BBC (2019) *Whorlton Hall: hospital 'abused' vulnerable adults.* Available at: www.bbc.co.uk/news/health-48367071 (accessed 2 January 2022).

Byrnes, K., Hamilton, S., McGeechan, G.J. *et al.* (2019) Attitudes and perceptions of people with a learning disability, family carers, and paid care workers towards cancer screening programmes in the United Kingdom: A qualitative systematic review and meta-aggregation. *Psycho-Oncology*, **23(3)**: 475–84.

Cumella, S. and Martin, D. (2000) *Secondary Healthcare for People with a Learning Disability: a report completed for the Department of Health.* British Institute of Learning Disabilities.

Department of Health (1995) *The Health of the Nation: a strategy for people with learning disabilities.* DH.

Department of Health (2012) *Transforming care: a national response to Winterbourne View Hospital*. Available at: https://assets.publishing.service.gov.uk/government/uploads/system/uploads/attachment_data/file/213215/final-report.pdf (accessed 2 January 2022).

Department of Health and Social Care (2019) *'Right to be heard': The Government's response to the consultation on learning disability and autism training for health and care staff*. Available at: https://assets.publishing.service.gov.uk/government/uploads/system/uploads/attachment_data/file/844356/autism-and-learning-disability-training-for-staff-consultation-response.pdf (accessed 2 January 2022).

Down's Syndrome Association (2021) *Annual health check information for GPs*. Available at: www.downs-syndrome.org.uk/wp-content/uploads/2021/04/Annual-Health-Check-2021.pdf (accessed 31 January 2022).

Epilepsy Action (2018) *Carers of people with epilepsy and a learning disability*. Available at: www.epilepsy.org.uk/info/carers/learning-disabilities (accessed 2 January 2022).

HEE (2021) *The Oliver McGowan Mandatory Training in Learning Disability and Autism*. Available at: www.hee.nhs.uk/our-work/learning-disability/oliver-mcgowan-mandatory-training-learning-disability-autism (accessed 2 January 2022).

Mencap (2018) *Concerns over lack of clinical training causing avoidable learning disability deaths*. Available at: www.mencap.org.uk/press-release/concerns-over-lack-clinical-training-causing-avoidable-learning-disability-deaths (accessed 2 January 2022).

Mencap (2021) *Mandatory learning disability and autism training*. Available at: www.mencap.org.uk/get-involved/campaign-mencap/treat-me-well/learning-disability-and-autism-training/mandatory (accessed 2 January 2022).

Neurotrauma Law Nexus (undated). *Neuroglossary*. Available at: www.neurolaw.com/neuroglossary/#d (accessed 2 January 2022).

NHS England (2014) *Winterbourne View – Time for Change* (also known as the *Bubb Report*). Available at: www.england.nhs.uk/wp-content/uploads/2014/11/transforming-commissioning-services.pdf (accessed 2 January 2022).

NHS Lothian (2020) *Hospital liaison service*. Available at: https://services.nhslothian.scot/LearningDisabilities/ClinicalServices/Pages/HospitalLiaisonService.aspx (accessed 2 January 2022).

NICE (2019) *Learning disability: care and support of people growing older* [QS187]. Available at: www.nice.org.uk/guidance/qs187/chapter/Quality-statement-5-Hospital-admissions (accessed 2 January 2022).

Northway, R., Rees, S., Davies, M. and Williams, S. (2017) Hospital passports, patient safety and person-centred care: A review of documents currently used for people with intellectual disabilities in the UK. *Journal of Clinical Nursing*, **26(23–24)**: 5160–8.

Public Health England (2018) *Learning disabilities: applying All Our Health*. Available at: www.gov.uk/government/publications/learning-disability-applying-all-our-health/learning-disabilities-applying-all-our-health (accessed 2 January 2022).

Royal College of General Practitioners (undated) *Health checks for people with learning disabilities toolkit*. Available from www.rcgp.org.uk/clinical-and-research/resources/toolkits/health-check-toolkit.aspx (accessed 2 January 2022).

RESOURCES

Core Capabilities Framework for Supporting People with a Learning Disability. Available at: https://skillsforhealth.org.uk/wp-content/uploads/2020/11/Learning-Disability-Framework-Oct-2019.pdf (accessed 2 January 2022).

Core Capabilities Framework for Supporting Autistic People. Available at: https://skillsforhealth.org.uk/wp-content/uploads/2020/11/Autism-Capabilities-Framework-Oct-2019.pdf (accessed 2 January 2022).

Chapter 6
Learning disability and consent to treatment

AIMS AND LEARNING OUTCOMES

The aims of this chapter are to:

- Define and discuss what consent is

- Discuss the issue of implied consent

- Highlight and discuss the contents of the Mental Capacity Act (MCA) 2005

- Highlight and discuss the nurse's role in consent and the applications of the MCA in relation to caring for someone who has a learning disability.

By the end of this chapter you will be able to:

- Discuss what consent is and is not

- Describe the contents of the Mental Capacity Act 2005

- Discuss how the MCA can be applied to those with a learning disability within a hospital setting.

SCENARIO 6.1

Marcel, a young man with Down's syndrome, arrives at the local Accident & Emergency (Casualty) department where Hanif works as a student nurse. Marcel was involved in a road traffic accident and, as a result, sustained a broken arm and leg. Marcel, who is unconscious, is accompanied by his sister Ziva who has Asperger's syndrome / high-functioning autism.

6.1 Introduction

Consent to treatment, indeed consent to any form of nursing, medical or social intervention, is a very complex issue and involves a wide range of professional, philosophical, legal and ethical questions and concerns. Registered nurses and other healthcare professionals will, in the course of a normal working day, have to assist patients or service users to make a myriad choices and decisions encompassing much of their daily lives whilst in their care. On occasion they may even have to either decide or contribute to the decision to provide nursing input if the patient is unable to decide for him- or herself. This may be for a wide range of reasons, including being unconscious, intoxicated through alcohol or other 'recreational' drugs or being in severe physical, mental or emotional pain. This is to be expected.

Likewise, nursing and other care staff are likely to encounter and work with people who have a learning disability who, due to their learning disability, will need extra support in making choices and decisions.

6.2 What is consent?

Issues of consent can be a legal minefield. For example, what do we mean by the following:

- What is the meaning of consent?
- Consent to and for what?
- Consent by whom?
- Consent for whom?

These are all valid and relevant questions and a lot of discussion by and between ethicists, philosophers, lawyers, nursing and medical practitioners, and patients / service users has taken place over the years in order to attempt to answer these questions, questions and answers which have had major implications and consequences for both patients / service users and hands-on clinical staff.

So, what is consent? Put simply:

> Consent refers to the provision of approval or agreement between two or more people or between a person and an organisation, particularly and especially after thoughtful consideration, for an action to take place.

According to the Oxford English Dictionary, consent is "the voluntary agreement to or acquiescence by one person in what another person proposes or desires".

In other words, say Hobden and Mills (2008), within a healthcare setting:

> *"consent is permission by a patient or service user for health care professionals to touch, question, examine or deliver care to the patient or service user".*

The RCN (2017), whilst not providing a 'dictionary definition' of consent, does stress its importance in the provision of any healthcare intervention or interaction in any healthcare setting.

Consent can be verbal, gestural or written. Without such consent, any form of nursing, medical or social care intervention risks being considered a form of abuse.

For consent to be valid, the following criteria must be met:

- The consent has to be based on sufficient relevant and accessible information
- be voluntarily given and not by coercion
- and given by somebody who is capable of giving consent.

For Marcel our scenario patient, as for everyone else, information must be in a format and manner that can be readily understood. Such information could be presented as:

- visual images such as pictures, line drawings and photos
- spoken words using simple language and short sentences
- leaflets, again using simple language and short and simple sentence structure
- sign language such as Makaton
- a combination of these.

Information requirements and the ways that information is presented are likely to change over time and even from situation to situation.

Consent must be voluntary. This is particularly relevant when a person is vulnerable or placed in a vulnerable position, such as having a learning disability, experiencing mental ill-health, experiencing acute pain, being the recipient of bad news, being under the influence of alcohol or other recreational drugs or being unconscious. Care must be taken to ensure that consent is not obtained through coercion, bullying or the offering of inducements. Such a situation is likely to be seen as abusive and any 'consent' obtained is likely to be invalid.

Those with a learning disability (such as Marcel) and/or those with a mental health issue must not be deemed unable to give or withhold consent purely on the grounds of their learning disability or mental health issue. There are strict criteria for assessing a person's mental capacity and ability to give consent; more about this later.

Remember, those who give consent for any form of medical or nursing intervention also have the legal and moral right to refuse to give consent or to withdraw consent at any time for a good reason, a bad reason or for no reason at all, and this right must be upheld.

6.3 Forms of consent

6.3.1 Express consent

Express consent is where the patient articulates consent to a proposed course of action; this can be verbally, through gestures or in writing. In a more structured setting such as pre-operation, consent is usually recorded in writing using a pre-printed form. However, a problem may arise where there is a dispute between the patient and the care professional around the contents of any verbal consent. Here, what was said may come down to the patient's word against that of the healthcare professional (Hobden and Mills, 2008). Never forget that the patient has a right to refuse to give consent or to withdraw consent once consent has been given.

In purely legal terms, there is no real difference between written and verbal consent and one form is not superior to the other (Hobden and Mills, 2008). However, the more complex the medical or surgical procedure, the more complex the information that the patient needs and thus the consent that is required.

6.3.2 Implied consent

Implied consent is no consent at all: discuss.

PAUSE FOR THOUGHT 6.2

Marcel is now conscious and has been admitted to the ward on which Sally works as a part-time senior staff nurse. During the morning drug round Sally approaches Marcel without saying anything about medication and he holds his hand out. Is this Marcel consenting to the receiving and taking of medication or is it learned behaviour?

Implied consent is where the patient's behaviour indicates that they are giving consent to whatever intervention is being proposed. This could include:

- Marcel holding out his hand when Sally approaches him with his medicines during a drug round
- a person arriving at the A&E department where their presence at the department implies consent to nursing and/or medical intervention
- a patient at a GP practice blood test clinic rolling their sleeve up in readiness for having a blood sample taken, although the GP or practice nurse may not have asked them to do so.

However, be very careful here. Consent, be it expressed or implied, must not be taken as a blanket permission that covers all forms of treatment, intervention or procedure throughout the patient's stay at the hospital, healthcare clinic or GP surgery. If Marcel arrives on the ward where Sally works with an overnight bag, Sally and her colleagues must not take this as implied consent for major invasive surgical procedures – unless, of course, he is booked in for such procedures. Again, consent is not a single one-off event but is a dynamic phenomenon and process and must be sought and given for each intervention or treatment that is proposed.

One risk with implied consent is that healthcare professionals may make assumptions about the patient's willingness to consent based upon their current or previous actions or behaviours. Therefore, it is advisable to always check with the patient as to whether or not they are giving consent.

6.4 Mental Capacity Act 2005

According to McIver (2006), the Mental Capacity Act (MCA) 2005 (originally the Mental Incapacity Bill), which affects everyone over the age of 16 years whose mental capacity is in doubt, is "one of the most controversial pieces of legislation that relates to people with a learning disability". Controversial issues regarding mental capacity, decision-making and consent could include sexuality (Rowlands, 2011) and Covid-19 (Mental Capacity Law and Policy, 2020). Mental capacity, in relation to the MCA, refers to the ability of the individual to make a decision about a number of aspects of their life, such as the ability to understand information and give fully informed consent, withdraw or withhold such consent. This would be the case not only in any healthcare setting but in other areas of life as well.

In its introductory paragraph, the MCA states that it is:

"… an Act to make new provision relating to persons who lack capacity; to establish a superior court of record called the Court of Protection in place of the office of the Supreme Court called by that name; to make provision in connection with the Convention on the International Protection of Adults signed at the Hague on 13th January 2000; and for connected purposes"

(www.legislation.gov.uk/ukpga/2005/9/introduction)

So, how would the Mental Capacity Act 2005 impact upon Marcel throughout his stay at hospital following his road traffic accident? Remember that when Marcel first entered the hospital following his accident, he was unconscious and that when he was transferred to Sally's ward he was conscious. Therefore, his mental capacity, his ability to understand information and give, withhold or withdraw informed consent has changed, and will change over time.

The stated aims of the Mental Capacity Act 2005 are to provide a statutory framework that will empower and protect vulnerable people who are unable to make their own decisions and to make clear who can take decisions on behalf of another person and in what circumstances.

McIver suggests that:

"Individual care plans will have to conform to the principles of the Act, demonstrating that service users have either been involved in decisions about their care, or that they have been assessed as lacking the capacity to do so and that the decisions made are in their best interests."

(McIver, 2006, p. 154)

6.4.1 What the Act says

The Mental Capacity Act 2005 is in three separate parts:

- **Part 1** contains 44 separate sections and focuses on people who may not possess mental capacity to make decisions or may have fluctuating ability.
- **Part 2** focuses on the Court of Protection and the Public Guardian.
- **Part 3** deals with miscellaneous and general issues.
- There are an additional eleven 'Schedules' which focus on specific issues such as deprivation of liberty and lasting power of attorney.

It is likely that Part 1 of the MCA will be the most applicable to those who engage on a daily basis with people who have a learning disability. The three boxes below are direct quotes from the Act.

Part 1: Section 1 of the MCA: The principles

This introduces the five key principles that apply throughout the MCA:

- A person must be assumed to have capacity unless it is established that he lacks capacity.
- A person is not to be treated as unable to make a decision [such as to give, refuse or withdraw consent] unless all practicable steps to help him to do so have been taken without success.
- A person is not to be treated as unable to make a decision merely because he makes an unwise decision.
- An act done, or decision made, under this Act for or on behalf of a person who lacks capacity must be done, or made, in his best interests.
- Before the act is done, or the decision is made, regard must be had to whether the purpose for which it is needed can be as effectively achieved in a way that is less restrictive of the person's rights and freedom of action.

(www.legislation.gov.uk/ukpga/2005/9/section/1)

Part 1: Section 2 of the MCA: People who lack capacity

1. For the purposes of this Act, a person lacks capacity in relation to a matter if at the material time he is unable to make a decision for himself in relation to the matter because of an impairment of, or a disturbance in the functioning of, the mind or brain.
2. It does not matter whether the impairment or disturbance is permanent or temporary.
3. A lack of capacity cannot be established merely by reference to –
    a. a person's age or appearance, or
    b. a condition of his, or an aspect of his behaviour, which might lead others to make unjustified assumptions about his capacity.
4. In proceedings under this Act or any other enactment, any question whether a person lacks capacity within the meaning of this Act must be decided on the balance of probabilities.
5. No power which a person ("D") may exercise under this Act is exercisable in relation to a person under 16
    (a) in relation to a person who lacks capacity, or
    (b) where D reasonably thinks that a person lacks capacity.

(www.legislation.gov.uk/ukpga/2005/9/section/2)

McIver (2006) suggests that, under Section 2, the individual patient, such as Marcel, does not have to prove that he or she has mental capacity, no more than under the English justice system a person has to prove his or her innocence. Again, each assessment of Marcel's capacity to make decisions must be time- and issue-specific. By this is meant that an assessment of capacity must be done every time that a decision has to be made and for every decision.

Section 3 of the MCA: Inability to make decisions

1. For the purposes of section 2, a person is unable to make a decision for himself if he is unable –
   (a) to understand the information relevant to the decision,
   (b) to retain that information,
   (c) to use or weigh that information as part of the process of making the decision, or
   (d) to communicate his decision (whether by talking, using sign language or any other means).

2. A person is not to be regarded as unable to understand the information relevant to a decision if he is able to understand an explanation of it given to him in a way that is appropriate to his circumstances (using simple language, visual aids or any other means).

3. The fact that a person is able to retain the information relevant to a decision for a short period only does not prevent him from being regarded as able to make the decision.

4. The information relevant to a decision includes information about the reasonably foreseeable consequences of –
   (a) deciding one way or another, or
   (b) failing to make the decision.

(www.legislation.gov.uk/ukpga/2005/9/section/3)

However, McIver (2006) suggests that "failure alone to understand the relevant information is not sufficient to demonstrate a lack of mental capacity"; Marcel is therefore not to be treated as unable to make decisions regarding his medical and nursing care simply because he makes an unwise decision. Section 4 will be highlighted in the next section.

There are a number of important sections of the MCA that will impact upon nursing care and support for Marcel and others with a learning disability whilst accessing healthcare:

- Sections 9–14 and 22–23: Lasting powers of attorney. This is when a person appoints and gives legal authority to another person to act in his or her best interests in relation to personal, health, social or financial welfare. This other person can be a family member or friend;
- Sections 24–26: Advance decisions to refuse treatment. This relates to a person's right to refuse, in advance, any nursing or medical intervention or treatment.

6.5 Assessing mental capacity

PAUSE FOR THOUGHT 6.3

Marcel arrives, unconscious, in the A&E department where Hanif works. Marcel is, consequently, unable to make any decisions about his nursing and medical care. However, he still needs to be assessed and treated. How would Hanif assess Marcel's mental capacity and Marcel's ability to make decisions? What does he do if Marcel cannot make such decisions?

Marcel is unable to offer, withhold or withdraw consent to nursing and medical intervention and treatment when he arrives at the A&E department and it would be wrong to wait until he regains consciousness and his decision-making ability before offering such care. Hanif would have to act in Marcel's best interests in order to safeguard his life. Consequently, Hanif may well be involved in discussions around assessing Marcel's mental capacity under direct supervision of the senior nurse on duty. Such discussions may include the following:

- Does Marcel have either a permanent or temporary impairment of, or disturbance in, the functioning of the mind or brain?
- Although unconscious and thus meeting this criterion, is this unconsciousness sufficient to imply that Marcel lacks the capacity to make a particular decision?

This is known as the 'two-stage test for capacity'.

The answer to this second question can be determined by considering whether, after being given all help and support to make the decision, Marcel cannot do the following:

1. Understand and absorb basic information relevant to the decision to be made
2. Retain the information long enough to process it
3. Weigh up the advantages and disadvantages against his value system
4. Communicate his decision.

Marcel is unconscious and thus unable to do any of these things, so he would be considered to lack capacity. However, if he is able to do all of these things, he may be assessed as having capacity to make his own decisions. This will be important when he regains consciousness, and even if information has to be given in alternative and simple communication forms and/or is retained for very short periods of time, this is not to be seen as meaning that he lacks capacity.

6.5.1 Best interests

As part of this discussion around capacity, a discussion that has to be ongoing given that Marcel is likely to regain consciousness, the issue of 'best interests' must be highlighted (see 'Section 4' box below). Again, Hanif, being a student nurse who is on duty at the time, is likely to be part of this discussion but will not lead it, as this would be the role of more senior and experienced nursing and medical colleagues. Again, decisions around what is and is not in Marcel's best interests are likely to be as a result of team discussions, with the nurse manager and/or doctor taking the ultimate responsibility for such decisions.

> **Part 1: Section 4 of the MCA: Best interests**
> 1. In determining for the purposes of this Act what is in a person's best interests, the person making the determination must not make it merely on the basis of –
>   (a) the person's age or appearance, or
>   (b) a condition of his, or an aspect of his behaviour, which might lead others to make unjustified assumptions about what might be in his best interests.
> 2. The person making the determination must consider all the relevant circumstances and, in particular, take the following steps.

3. He must consider –
    (a) whether it is likely that the person will at some time have capacity in relation to the matter in question, and
    (b) if it appears likely that he will, when that is likely to be.
4. He must, so far as reasonably practicable, permit and encourage the person to participate, or to improve his ability to participate, as fully as possible in any act done for him and any decision affecting him.
5. Where the determination relates to life-sustaining treatment he must not, in considering whether the treatment is in the best interests of the person concerned, be motivated by a desire to bring about his death.
6. He must consider, so far as is reasonably ascertainable –
    (a) the person's past and present wishes and feelings (and, in particular, any relevant written statement made by him when he had capacity),
    (b) the beliefs and values that would be likely to influence his decision if he had capacity, and
    (c) the other factors that he would be likely to consider if he were able to do so.
7. He must take into account, if it is practicable and appropriate to consult them, the views of –
    (a) anyone named by the person as someone to be consulted on the matter in question or on matters of that kind,
    (b) anyone engaged in caring for the person or interested in his welfare,
    (c) any donee of a lasting power of attorney granted by the person, and
    (d) any deputy appointed for the person by the court, as to what would be in the person's best interests and, in particular, as to the matters mentioned in subsection (6).
8. The duties imposed by subsections (1) to (7) also apply in relation to the exercise of any powers which –
    (a) are exercisable under a lasting power of attorney, or
    (b) are exercisable by a person under this Act where he reasonably believes that another person lacks capacity.
9. In the case of an act done, or a decision made, by a person other than the court, there is sufficient compliance with this section if (having complied with the requirements of subsections (1) to (7)) he reasonably believes that what he does or decides is in the best interests of the person concerned.
10. "Life-sustaining treatment" means treatment which in the view of a person providing health care for the person concerned is necessary to sustain life.
11. "Relevant circumstances" are those –
    (a) of which the person making the determination is aware, and
    (b) which it would be reasonable to regard as relevant.

(www.legislation.gov.uk/ukpga/2005/9/section/4)

The basic rule here is to act in the least restrictive way possible under the circumstances. Remember to ensure that any decision made in another person's best interests regarding his or her care follows organisational policies and protocols, is made with the agreement of all stakeholders and is recorded and documented thoroughly.

6.6 **The role of the nurse**

Let's recap a little.

Having been involved in a road traffic accident, Marcel arrives unconscious at A&E where Hanif works as a student nurse. Is Hanif required to seek Marcel's consent prior to providing nursing care?

Because he is unconscious, Marcel is unable to provide, refuse or withdraw consent (MCA Section 2:1). While this does not mean that Hanif can ride roughshod over what Marcel would have preferred had he been in a position to give consent, Hanif is permitted to provide emergency life-sustaining nursing care (Sections 1:3, 4:10). Hanif would not be guilty of assault as long as he acted in Marcel's best interests, in line with departmental policies and protocols and in good faith. In relation to Marcel's 'best interests', it is vital that all other people engaged in Marcel's care are involved in decision-making (Sections 4:6a–c, 7a–b). This must include: other nurses, doctors, Marcel's family and any advance statement that Marcel may have written. It is vital that any nursing care (and medical care for that matter) is arrived at through a consensus of professional and family views and opinion and must be recorded, along with the reasons for the interventions and the reasons why consent could not be given by Marcel. Marcel's level of consciousness and his ability to decide and consent must be reviewed regularly and acted upon (Section 4:3a–b).

Once Marcel has recovered consciousness and his pain and distress levels do not impede his decision-making and consent-giving abilities, then he must be encouraged to participate in nursing intervention decisions and consent (Section 4:4).

Because of Marcel's learning disability, Marcel is likely to need information presented to him in simpler ways that he is more likely to understand. Therefore, without being patronising or condescending to Marcel, Hanif should seek the assistance of those who work and live with him and, if possible, the learning disability liaison nurse on how to present information to Marcel in ways that he can understand.

PAUSE FOR THOUGHT 6.4

Marcel has now been transferred to the general medical ward. It is the evening 'drug round' and Marcel refuses his medication. Is it right to try to disguise his medicine by mixing it with his food? Discuss.

In times gone by, it was fairly common practice to administer medicine by mixing it with food. However, Marcel has a right to make decisions, in this case to refuse to give consent to accept his evening medication, for a good reason, a bad reason or for no reason at all; having a learning disability is not grounds for believing that Marcel is unable to give consent (Section 2:3b). The nurse working with Marcel should try to find out why Marcel is refusing his medication and work around this. It could be that Marcel does not like the nurse who is administering the medication, that he has friends or family visiting, that he is tired, or for many other reasons. If it is possible, in the case of the former, the nurse working with Marcel should ask a colleague who

Marcel likes, to administer the medication or come back at a later time to administer the medication. The same applies to any other forms of nursing intervention such as meeting his personal hygiene needs (washing, dressing, toileting, shaving, etc.). As Marcel is likely to be anxious and frightened as a result of having been hit by a car and being in a strange and alien environment, the nurse working with Marcel should try to enlist the help of his family and the learning disability liaison nurse.

6.7 Conclusion

Consent and the mental capacity to give, refuse to give or withdraw such consent have been highly complex and thorny legal, philosophical, ethical, nursing and medical issues for decades. This is true not only for those with a learning disability but for many other patient or service user groups such as the elderly, young teenagers and those who experience mental health issues. Despite the existence of the Mental Capacity Act 2005, issues around consent and mental capacity are likely to persist for the foreseeable future. However, Marcel's rights to refuse and withdraw consent need to be respected, promoted and safeguarded in order to provide high-quality care and to avoid any accusation of abuse.

CHAPTER SUMMARY

Key points to take away from *Chapter 6*:
- ☑ Those with a learning disability have the right to refuse and withdraw consent to treatment and interventions for a good reason, a bad reason or for no reason at all.
- ☑ Consent can be expressed or implied.
- ☑ For consent to be valid, the following criteria must be met. The consent has to be based on sufficient relevant information, voluntary and given by somebody who is capable of giving consent.
- ☑ The stated aims of the Mental Capacity Act 2005 are to provide a statutory framework that will empower and protect vulnerable people who are unable to make their own decisions and to make clear who can take decisions on behalf of another person and in what circumstances.
- ☑ The Mental Capacity Act encompasses such issues as consent, best interest, lasting power of attorney, deprivation of liberty and courts of protection.

Questions

Question 6.1	What is meant by the word *'consent'*?
Question 6.2	What is needed for consent to be valid?
Question 6.3	What is 'implied consent' and is it legally valid?
Question 6.4	How would you assess mental capacity?
Question 6.5	Can a family member or care professional give consent for another person?
Question 6.6	What is meant by 'best interests'?
Question 6.7	What are the key principles of Sections 1, 2 and 3 of the Mental Capacity Act 2005?

REFERENCES

Hobden, A. and Mills, S. (2008) 'Consent and capacity'. In Clark, L. and Griffiths, P. (eds) *Learning Disability and Other Intellectual Impairments: meeting needs through health services*. John Wiley & Sons.

McIver, M. (2006) 'Legislation and learning disability'. In Peate, I. and Fearns, D. (eds) *Caring for People with Learning Disabilities*. John Wiley & Sons.

Mental Capacity Act 2005. Available at: www.legislation.gov.uk/ukpga/2005/9/introduction (accessed 3 January 2022).

Mental Capacity Law and Policy (2020) *COVID-19 and the MCA 2005*. Available at: www.mentalcapacitylawandpolicy.org.uk/resources-2/covid-19-and-the-mca-2005 (accessed 3 January 2022).

Rowlands, S. (2011) Learning disability and contraceptive decision-making. *BMJ Sexual & Reproductive Health*, **37**: 173–8. Available at: https://srh.bmj.com/content/37/3/173 (accessed 3 January 2022).

Royal College of Nursing (2017) Principles of consent: guidance for nursing staff. *British Journal of Healthcare Assistants*, **11(10)**: 498–502.

Chapter 7
Learning disability and mental health

AIMS AND LEARNING OUTCOMES

The aims of this chapter are to:

- Investigate the meaning of mental health from a clinical and service user perspective

- Explore the various forms of mental health problems

- Highlight the prevalence of mental health issues within those with a learning disability

- Explore the various forms of therapeutic intervention that are available when working with those who have a learning disability who also experience mental health issues.

By the end of this chapter you will be able to reflect upon and discuss:

- The meaning of mental health

- The various forms of mental ill-health

- The prevalence and incidence of mental health problems within those with a learning disability

- The availability and value of a range of therapeutic and management strategies

- The application of these strategies to those with a learning disability.

7.1 Introduction

Many years ago it was thought that those with a learning disability were unable to develop mental illnesses or mental health problems, as to do so requires a certain level of mental, cognitive and intellectual development, ability and functioning. It was believed that those with a learning disability may not have the intellectual or cognitive level 'needed' to experience mental illness (Smiley, 2005). However, anyone who works with those with a learning disability within a hospital, a residential or a community setting will be very much aware that those with a learning disability can indeed experience the same mental health issues that are prevalent within wider society (Barber, 2011). Again, it could be argued that there is much misunderstanding within society at large, a lack of understanding that is reflected in the nursing profession (Priest and Gibbs, 2004) with regard to the differences between mental health and learning disabilities, with some people believing that these are the same thing. Maloret (2006) suggests that this lack of understanding may be a result of a lack of education in the area of mental health and learning disabilities.

It is likely that as a nurse working in a general hospital, GP practice, health centre or community nursing team you will meet and work with people who have both a learning disability and who are experiencing a mental health problem.

7.2 **What is mental health?**

PAUSE FOR THOUGHT 7.1

Mental health, mental illness, psycho, schizo, depressive, nuts, bonkers, mad…. What's in a name?

Learning disability is not the same thing as a mental illness or mental health condition. Having a learning disability is not the same thing as having clinical depression, bipolar disorder or schizophrenia, for example. Sometimes, it is said that a person with a learning disability may have a 'dual diagnosis'. By this is meant having both a learning disability and a mental health problem. This can sometimes appear confusing, as the term 'dual diagnosis' can also refer to those who experience mental health problems and who use/misuse drugs such as cannabis, cocaine, heroin or alcohol. Those with a learning disability are not immune to such drug use and therefore both senses of the term 'dual diagnosis' can apply. Due to a possible 'overlap' of behavioural signs and symptoms (Maloret, 2006), misdiagnosis of mental health problems within those with a learning disability can sometimes happen, with mental health problems being dismissed as being an aspect of what it is to have a learning disability. So, what is mental health and is mental health the same as mental illness?

It may be helpful here to look at the word 'health'. Health is both an absence of illness and the optimum 'performance' of the body. Therefore, mental health could be seen as both an absence of mental illness and the 'optimum performance' of the person's mental and cognitive faculties and mind, whereas mental illness could be seen as any mental health condition that has a negative effect on how an individual thinks, feels and behaves. The World Health Organization in its Constitution defines health as 'being a state of complete physical, mental and social well-being and not merely the absence of disease or infirmity' (WHO, 2020).

Mental illness could be argued to have a number of definitions and meanings, including:

A mental health problem, as defined by the American Psychiatric Association, is: "a clinically significant behavioural or psychological syndrome or pattern that is associated with present distress or disability or with a significantly increased risk of suffering death, pain, disability or loss of freedom" (APA, 2013 (DSM-5)). Basically, this means that "a mental health problem exists when there is a change in a person's behaviour, thought processes or mood to the extent that day-to-day life is adversely affected" (Maloret, 2006).

Mental disorder: Taylor (2019) suggests that this term was defined by the Mental Health Act 1983 to cover all forms of mental illness and disability, including mental impairment and psychopathic disorder.

Mental illness: a category not defined by the Mental Health Act 1983 or any other mental health-related legislation and which is therefore left open to interpretation. However, mental illness could also be described as a term that is used to describe a number of disorders of the mind that affect the emotions, perceptions, reasoning or memory of the individual (Taylor, 2019).

Mental hygiene: "the science that deals with the development of healthy mental and emotional reactions" (Taylor, 2019). This term has also been used in the past to define or categorise mental illness. However, this term could have somewhat negative and unhelpful connotations regarding the moral standing of the person; whether the person who has and experiences a mental health issue is morally and socially 'unhygienic' or 'unclean'.

Again, the use of certain, often negative, language to define a person's mental state could allow the 'non-mentally ill' to exercise control and power over those who experience mental health problems or difficulties.

7.3 Forms of mental ill-health

Having briefly looked at a number of basic, if contrasting and even conflicting, definitions of mental health and mental illness, attention will now be shifted to highlight the various forms that mental ill-health can take. I am indebted to Mark Allen Publishing and the *British Journal of Healthcare Assistants* for their kind permission to include the following information from Barber (2011) in this section.

There are wide varieties and forms of mental ill-health which include the following:

Depression: Depression can be seen as "a morbid and long-lasting sadness or melancholy which may, or may not, be a symptom of an underlying psychiatric problem" (Taylor, 2019, p. 120). Causes of depression are likely to be numerous, and symptoms may include:
- persistent lowered mood for most of the day
- decreased interest, pleasure or non-engagement in previously enjoyed daily or weekly activities
- difficulty in sleeping
- significant weight gain or loss

- chronic feelings of being worthless, useless and a failure
- diminished ability to think, concentrate or make decisions
- thoughts of death, dying, self-harm or suicide.

Bipolar conditions: This used to be known as 'manic depression' and is characterised by a single or multiple episodes of dramatic and severe mood swings between the two extreme poles of severe mania and severe depression. Bipolar conditions are chronic and recurrent, with the manic phase sometimes requiring hospital admission and treatment.

Dementia: Dementia is a gradual but global and progressive death of brain cells leading to a gradual and irreversible decline in all areas of mental functioning, including memory, intellect, social judgement, personality, social skills / behaviour and physical skills. While dementia is usually associated with old age, it is not unheard of for symptoms to appear at any age.

Addictions: These are a persistent, compulsive dependence on a behaviour (such as sex, work, gambling or shopping) or substance such as alcohol or drugs.

Anxiety disorder: Anxiety is a normal part of what it is to be human; it is a normal aspect of human experiences. Anxiety conditions can be seen as an extreme anxiety response to certain memories, experiences or anticipated experiences and unwarranted worrying can either cause or trigger anxiety states. Physical and behavioural symptoms of anxiety may include:
- palpitations
- sweating and dry mouth
- elevated blood pressure
- fear, apprehension, sense of impending doom, terror or dread
- altered sleep patterns
- irritability
- panic.

Attention deficit and hyperactivity disorder (ADHD): ADHD is characterised by abnormal levels of inattention, hyperactivity, or their combination. The person must present with the following: inattention (usually has difficulty maintaining attention in activities) and hyperactivity / impulsivity (is often 'on the go' or often acts as if 'driven by a motor').

Obsessive–compulsive disorder (OCD): An obsession is a persistent, often intrusive and unwanted thought, emotion or behaviour that the person cannot ignore. A compulsion is a behavioural manifestation of the obsessive thought. Such behavioural manifestations could include the performance of a repetitious, uncontrollable but seemingly purposeful act or ritual, such as the constant washing of hands, constant checking to see if the lights are turned off or the front door is closed and locked.

Schizophrenia: Major symptoms could include:
- delusional thinking and perceptions
- auditory hallucinations or 'thought echo'

- broadcasting, withdrawal or insertion of thoughts into a person's head
- thought disorder, 'word salad', loosened associations
- obsessive preoccupation with fantasy and esoteric ideas
- showing less interest, enthusiasm or emotion than usual
- inappropriate behaviour.

Borderline personality disorder (BPD): This is a collection of personality traits that underpin certain groups of behaviours, including:
- frantic efforts to avoid real or imagined abandonment
- a pattern of unstable / intense interpersonal relationships
- markedly and persistently unstable self-image or sense of self
- potentially self-damaging impulsivity
- recurrent suicidal behaviour
- chronic feelings of emptiness
- inappropriate, intense anger or inability to control anger
- short-lived stress-related paranoid thoughts.

7.4 **Prevalence**

Having briefly looked at the varied forms of mental health issues, problems and conditions that many people can experience throughout their lives, we will now consider how prevalent these issues are. People with learning disabilities are likely to experience the complete spectrum of mental health problems, with higher prevalence than in those without learning disabilities, as can be seen from *Table 7.1*.

The Foundation for People with Learning Disabilities suggests that "children and young people with learning disabilities are much more likely than others to live in poverty, to have few friends and to have additional long-term health problems and disabilities such as epilepsy and sensory impairments. All these factors are positively associated with mental health problems" (FPLD, 2020).

Table 7.1 *Prevalence of mental health conditions in the UK*

Mental health conditions	Those with a learning disability (1–1.5 million)	General UK population (around 65 million)
All mental health problems	25–40% (36% of children and adolescents)	25% (8% of children and adolescents)
Schizophrenia	3%	1%
Depression	12.5%	2.8%
Bipolar	1.5%	1–2%
Anxiety disorder	16.7%	8–12%
OCD	2.5–9.4%	1.2%

(continued)

Table 7.1 *(continued)*

Mental health conditions	Those with a learning disability (1–1.5 million)	General UK population (around 65 million)
Dementia	21.6% (those with Down's syndrome are at particularly high risk of developing dementia, with an age of onset 30–40 years younger than the general population)	5.7%
Autism spectrum conditions	Around 35%	1–1.1%

Sources: Smiley (2005); Devine *et al.* (2010); FPLD (2020); Mencap (2021).

According to the Foundation for People with Learning Disabilities, 10–15% of people with a learning disability are also likely to exhibit 'challenging behaviours' (aggression, destruction, self-injury and others) with age-specific prevalence peaking between the ages of 20 and 49.

However, caution must be exercised in a number of areas.

Although autism is a condition recognised by the American Psychiatric Association in its DSM-5 (APA, 2013), it is not a mental health condition in itself, even if many of those on the autism spectrum are likely to experience mental health issues at a higher level than in the general population. Autism is more a developmental than a mental health condition. However, many people who are on the autism spectrum, particularly those with Asperger's syndrome or high-functioning autism, will not experience either a learning disability or a mental health issue and will thus fall between the cracks of service provision that may be targeted at those with a learning disability and/or a mental health condition but may not accept or understand that those with high-functioning autism/Asperger's may also need help and support.

Whilst 'challenging behaviour' such as aggression, antisocial behaviour and self-harm can often be a sign or symptom of a mental health issue, it is not a mental health condition in itself.

The reader should be aware of, and exercise caution in potentially pathologising normal or near-normal human responses to normal life experiences as mental health issues. One such example is the inclusion of bereavement as a potential mental health condition in DSM-5.

While anecdotal evidence suggests a link between mental ill-health and learning disabilities, actual prevalence in percentage terms of mental health problems in people with a learning disability can prove to be somewhat elusive. In other words, according to Barber (2011), it is uncertain how many people with a learning disability will also experience a mental health problem. Even Mencap, in response to a personal emailed enquiry from the author, does not hold such data and was thus unaware of prevalence or comparison rates in terms of those without a learning disability. Although this was still the situation towards the end of 2021, Mencap (2021) suggests that there are links between learning disabilities and mental health issues, stating that those with a learning disability are at vastly increased risk of developing a mental health issue, whilst not developing this argument further by providing actual statistics.

There are "lies, damned lies and statistics" (a phrase mistakenly attributed by the American writer Mark Twain to the 19th century British Prime Minister Benjamin Disraeli and popularised in the USA by Twain, amongst others)! Beware of misusing or accepting the simple statistics given in this chapter and throughout the book at face value.

7.5 The role of the nurse

SCENARIO 7.1

Tariq is a 48-year-old gentleman with Down's syndrome who experiences severe anxiety and hears voices. Following a minor stroke at the care home where he lives, Tariq has been admitted to the general medical ward where Hanif works as a student. As Hanif has previously indicated an interest in mental health issues, he has been asked to assist in Tariq's care during his stay on the ward.

Although learning disability and mental ill-health are not the same conditions, those with a learning disability are statistically more likely to experience a mental health problem than those who do not have a learning disability, and Tariq is no different.

Reading Tariq's notes, Hanif finds that Tariq, although admitted to the hospital ward following a minor stroke, has a number of underlying mental health issues which have no connection to the stroke. According to his notes, Tariq experiences severe anxiety issues and hears voices. Observing and interacting with Tariq, Hanif comes to believe that he is also experiencing depression. What are Hanif's roles in Tariq's care?

The nursing process (assess, plan, implement and evaluate) may be a useful tool that would aid Hanif when working with Tariq. However, it must be kept in mind that Tariq may not be on the ward long enough for Hanif to carry out a thorough and in-depth assessment and planning.

7.5.1 Assess

Initially, Hanif's role is to become fully aware of Tariq's mental health history and how the mental health issues impact upon Tariq's daily life. Hanif needs to understand what 'normal' behaviour and mood means for Tariq. This may sound strange but be aware that everyone has a slightly different take on what 'normal' is: what is 'normal' in terms of mood and behaviour for one person may not be 'normal' for someone else. Also, what may be a problem in terms of mental health behaviour for one person may not be a problem for another. Hanif also needs to assess how Tariq's mental health and moods may be affected by the stroke. Hanif should be able to ascertain this baseline data through a combination of:

- interacting with, observing, talking with and listening to Tariq
- reading Tariq's nursing and medical notes
- talking to those who are significant in Tariq's life, such as his family and his support workers
- seeking the advice of the learning disability liaison nurse and visiting mental health nurse, psychologist and psychiatrist.

Communication will play a vital role in meeting Tariq's holistic needs whilst on the ward. This includes communicating with colleagues, family and, above all, Tariq. It must be remembered that connecting psychologically and emotionally with Tariq through communication and interaction is a basic human need and right and that mental ill-health is not catching! Communicating with Tariq may make it easier and less intrusive to observe for any subtle changes in his mental state, his mood and his behaviour.

7.5.2 Plan

There are a number of therapeutic forms that could be helpful to Tariq in managing his mental health problems.

Pharmacotherapy: Drugs such as chlorpromazine and haloperidol (management of psychosis), lithium carbonate (management of bipolar conditions), nitrazepam (night-time sedation), fluoxetine (management of depression) and diazepam and lorazepam (management of anxiety disorders) could be helpful here. These drugs have been used for many decades to manage behavioural and mood disorders in those with a learning disability. It is likely that as Tariq experiences auditory hallucinations and severe anxiety issues, he would already be using medication to manage his symptoms. Hanif's role is to encourage Tariq in continuing his medicine regime whilst he is in hospital, to answer any questions that Tariq may have about his medication and to monitor, report and record any drug benefits and side-effects that Tariq may be experiencing. However, Hanif may need to be aware of the possibility of using pharmacotherapy as forms of chemical restraint, and challenge this use. The role of Hanif's course lecturers is to foster this ability to question and challenge ideas, attitudes and practices, within certain limits.

Talking therapies: Talking therapies, including cognitive behavioural therapies (CBT), dialectic behaviour therapy (DBT), psychodynamic therapies, humanistic therapies, and support and information, give people the chance to explore their thoughts and feelings and the effect they have on their behaviour and mood. Devine (2018) suggests that talking therapies may be a useful tool when working with those who have a mild learning disability or high-functioning autism and that such talking therapies should not be refused simply on the grounds of the patient or service user having a learning disability.

Complementary therapies: These will include hypnotherapy, reiki, meditation, acupressure, acupuncture and prayer or other spiritual exercises. Although used for centuries in China, India and Japan, their effectiveness with those with a learning disability is under-researched and under-tested and they must therefore be used with great caution. However, a wide range of complementary therapies is becoming more popular in the UK and as many of these forms of therapy rely to a large extent on holistic human connectedness and compassion, they can rarely be unsafe.

Just because there may not be much research evidence to support a particular form of therapeutic management or treatment of mental health issues in people with a learning disability, as is the case with complementary and, to a lesser extent, talking therapies, this does not mean that these should not be considered. However, extreme caution must be exercised in suggesting the use of untried and unresearched therapeutic interventions, and Hanif would seek guidance from the hospital's learning disability liaison nurse and his course tutors and module lecturers.

Any resultant care plan must be centred around the mental health needs of the individual (in this example, Tariq) and be tailored to meet those needs. Whilst it may be tempting to write a care plan that offers 'quick fixes' in terms of goals and outcomes, given that Tariq will only be on the ward a relatively short time, any care plan needs to be measurable, realistic and achievable. There is no point in writing a care plan that cannot be achieved or is unrealistic given the existing resources that Hanif has at his disposal. Likewise, any care plan needs to have the active agreement and participation of all stakeholders, including all the relevant ward staff, as without such agreement and participation any care plan is doomed to failure and risks potentially harming Tariq.

Given the likely short time resource available to Hanif, an appropriate care plan must include post-discharge strategies which must include, with Tariq's consent, communicating and active cooperation with the staff at Tariq's care home and day care facilities and active communication and cooperating with community-based mental health services. Failure to plan for Tariq's discharge or leaving it to the last minute to carry out a discharge assessment and care plan risks failing Tariq and leaving the ward staff open to valid and legitimate complaints from Tariq, his care home staff and his family.

7.5.3 Implement

Any ward-based care plan that is devised for Tariq's ongoing mental health support would then be implemented by the multidisciplinary team including the ward staff, psychologists, mental health teams and Tariq. This must include preparations for a handover to Tariq's care home and community-based mental health team prior to Tariq's discharge.

7.5.4 Evaluate

Evaluation of any care plans or interventions that aim to support Tariq must be ongoing rather than seen as a 'one-off' event or activity. As Tariq's mental health issues have been long-standing and the time that he has spent on the ward short, it is unlikely that any evaluation will highlight any significant improvement in his mental state. However, there may be subtle changes that may indicate improvement in Tariq's anxiety and voice hearing, and these must be celebrated, recorded and fed into any pre-discharge assessment and care planning and future mental health assessment as the new mental health baseline.

7.6 Conclusion

Although learning disability and mental ill-health are not the same phenomenon, people with a learning disability are as likely as and indeed more likely than anyone else to experience mental health problems. Consequently, it is more than likely that, at some point in Hanif's nursing career, he will engage and support those with a dual diagnosis of learning disability and mental health issue. It is thus hoped that this chapter on learning disability and mental health will have aroused your interest in this fascinating area of work.

CHAPTER SUMMARY

Key points to take away from *Chapter 7*:
- ☑ Having a learning disability is not the same as having or experiencing a mental health problem.
- ☑ Those with a learning disability are as likely as, or even more likely to experience mental health issues than anyone else.
- ☑ A mental health problem is a clinically significant behavioural or psychological syndrome or pattern that is associated with present distress or disability or with a significantly increased risk of suffering death, pain, disability or loss of freedom. Mental health issues could include depression, schizophrenia, bipolar (manic depression), severe anxiety, addictions, obsession/compulsion, dementia, ADHD and borderline personality disorder.
- ☑ Forms of therapy could include medication, talking and listening to the patient and an increasing range of complementary therapies.

Questions

Question 7.1	What is mental health?
Question 7.2	How is mental ill-health different from learning disability?
Question 7.3	What are the forms of mental ill-health that a person with a learning disability may experience?
Question 7.4	What are the advantages and disadvantages to using the nursing process in relation to working with a patient with a learning disability and mental health issues?
Question 7.5	What methods or techniques are there for assessing and meeting, managing or treating a mental health condition?
Question 7.6	How would you evaluate the value and relevance of such methods and techniques for those with a learning disability?

REFERENCES

American Psychiatric Association (2013) *Diagnostic and Statistical Manual of Mental Disorders (DSM-5)*. APA.

Barber, C. (2011) Supporting mental health issues alongside learning disabilities. *British Journal of Healthcare Assistants*, **5(11)**: 548–52.

Devine, D. (2018) *Can cognitive behavioural therapy (CBT) work for those with learning disabilities?* Learning Disability Today. Available at: www.learningdisabilitytoday.co.uk/can-cognitive-behavioural-therapy-cbt-work-for-those-with-learning-disabilities (accessed 3 January 2022).

Devine, M., Taggart, L. and McLornian, P. (2010) Screening for mental health problems in adults with learning disabilities using the Mini PAS-ADD Interview. *British Journal of Learning Disabilities*, **36(4)**: 252–8.

Foundation for People with Learning Disabilities (2020) *Learning disability statistics: mental health problems*. Available at: www.learningdisabilities. org.uk/learning-disabilities/help-information/learning-disability-statistics-/187699 (accessed 3 January 2022).

Maloret, P. (2006) 'Mental health issues and adults with learning disabilities'. In Peate, I. and Fearns, D. (eds) *Caring for People with Learning Disabilities*. John Wiley & Sons.

Mencap (2021) *Mental health*. Available at: www.mencap.org.uk/learning-disability-explained/research-and-statistics/health/mental-health (accessed 3 January 2022).

Priest, H. and Gibbs, M. (2004) *Mental Health Care for People with Learning Disabilities*. Churchill Livingstone.

Smiley, E. (2005) Epidemiology of mental health problems in adults with learning disability: an update. *Advances in Psychiatric Treatment*, **11**: 214–22.

Taylor, J. (ed) (2019) *Baillière's Dictionary for Nurses and Healthcare Workers*, 27th edition. Elsevier.

World Health Organization (2020) *Basic Documents forty-ninth edition (including amendments adopted up to 31 May 2019)*. WHO.

FURTHER READING

Newton, M., Llewellyn, A. and Hayes, S. (2019) *The Care Process*. Lantern Publishing.

Chapter 8
Learning disability and forensic care

AIMS AND LEARNING OUTCOMES

The aims of this chapter are to:

- Briefly discuss the meaning of forensic services and care

- Tentatively present the numbers of those with a learning disability who are likely to come into contact with forensic services as either victims, perpetrators or witnesses to crime

- Chart a number of potential journeys through forensic services

- Present a number of ways in which those who encounter forensic services can be supported.

By the end of this chapter you will be able to discuss:

- What forensic services and care mean and involve in relation to those with a learning disability

- The statistics around people with a learning disability that are likely to come into contact with the forensic services, and the reasons for these contacts

- The impact of forensic care and services as experienced by three people with a learning disability

- A number of ways that those who come into contact with forensic services can be supported.

SCENARIO 8.1: VICTORIA

Victoria, a 20-year-old woman with a mild learning disability, has been arrested by the police for possessing a small amount of a 'Class B' substance (cannabis). This was not the first time that Victoria had come to the attention of the police. Previous encounters had been as a result of Victoria's 'antisocial behaviour' where she received a police caution. This is the first time that Victoria has been arrested for drug-related offences. Victoria lives with her parents who are finding it increasingly difficult to manage her behaviour.

SCENARIO 8.2: BRIAN

Brian, a 40-year-old with autism and a mild learning disability, has been arrested for sending sexually explicit video images of himself and written material over the internet (using a social networking site) to a 14-year-old girl. This offence was compounded by asking the girl to masturbate while watching the video images that he had sent her. Brian lives on his own but with multi-agency support. This was Brian's first offence.

SCENARIO 8.3: YASMIN

Yasmin, a 30-year-old with mild learning disability and autism who lives with her parents, has been subjected, on the grounds of her disability, to verbal and physical violence for the past three years by groups of youths and their parents who live on the same housing estate as she does. Yasmin arrives at her local police station after being kicked and punched by these youths.

8.1 Introduction

Evidence suggests that a person with a learning disability is as likely as any other person to come into contact with the various branches of the criminal justice system (Barber, 2011; see also *Section 8.3*). Nurses and healthcare professionals, whether working in forensic care services, more general care settings, or in the community, may well encounter crime victims or perpetrators who have a learning disability. This chapter provides an introduction to the ways that people with a learning disability who come into contact with forensic services can be supported, by means of our three scenarios.

8.2 What are forensic services?

There are three forms of forensic services. The first is the solving of crimes through scientific investigations. If one watches TV programmes such as the long-running British series *Silent Witness*, for example, one may already be aware of this aspect of forensic services. The second is the criminal justice system which includes the police, the courts and the probation services. Thirdly, forensic services also means a sub-branch of psychiatry that serves as the interface between the law, the various aspects of the criminal justice system such as the courts, prisons and the probation service, and psychiatry and residential or community mental health services (Burrow, 1993; RCN, 2019). This chapter will focus on the second and third aspects of the term 'forensic services'.

Kingdon (2009, p. 361) suggested that although there have been forensic services of sorts as far back as 1863, there is no nationally agreed definition of forensic services or the roles of those who work with them. Indeed, most, if not all, of the nineteenth and early twentieth century psychiatric institutions would have been what today would be called 'secure environments' and could thus be seen as 'forensic' in nature. Furthermore, an acceptable and universal definition of forensics and therefore what comprises forensic services is elusive (Kettles *et al.*, 2001; Baxter, 2002). However, Chaloner and Coffey (2000) did suggest that "forensic nursing is about the assessment, treatment and management of mentally disordered offenders across a spectrum of secure environments, including the community".

Put somewhat simply, the type of behaviour that would lead a person to access forensic services is any behaviour that would bring the individual into contact with the various arms of the criminal justice system, mainly the police, the courts and custodial services. This could include:

- arson
- theft
- burglary
- physical assault
- sexual assault (including rape)
- drug possession and supply
- hate/mate crimes (a 'mate crime' occurs when a person is harmed or taken advantage of by someone they thought was their friend)
- kidnapping
- 'conduct likely to cause a breach of the peace' such as fighting in public or rioting.

In all of these crime areas, the person with a learning disability can be a victim, a witness or a perpetrator.

In the context of forensics, learning disability is considered as a mental disorder and those with a learning disability as mentally disordered (University of Central Lancashire, 1999; Kearns, 2001). Kingdon (2009, p. 366) suggests that people who come to the attention of the forensic services are likely to be those who have a borderline to mild learning disability, a conclusion reinforced by Marshall-Tate *et al.* (2019).

The term 'forensic services' could be broken down into the following services, all of which nurses could potentially work in or come into contact with.

Prisons: Here, nurses will meet the physical and mental healthcare needs of prison inmates, regardless of whether the inmate has been previously diagnosed with a learning disability or mental health issue. For information and further reading on prison nursing see the Royal College of Nursing's (RCN) Nursing in Criminal Justice Services Forum (see *Further Reading*).

Secure settings: Again, nurses within secure settings, such as Rampton Hospital in Nottinghamshire, will meet the physical, mental and emotional needs of the service users within a holistic framework. Services at Rampton, for example, will include mental health, female services, learning disabilities and personality (including dangerous and severe) disorders.

Medium to low community-based secure settings: Medium security settings are those that provide a residential and therapeutic environment and service for those convicted of a crime but who present a serious but less immediate danger to others and have the potential to abscond. Low security settings are intended for those service users who present a less serious physical danger to others. Their security measures are intended to impede rather than prevent absconding, with greater reliance on staffing arrangements and less reliance on physical security measures.

Forensic psychiatry: This is a service that provides a bridge between mental health services and the criminal justice services.

8.3 Prevalence

It appears that large numbers of those who appear before the courts, both young people and adults, are likely to have a learning disability (Jacobson and Talbot, 2009). It is not known exactly how many people with a learning disability are likely to come into contact with the forensic services, be it as victims, witnesses or perpetrators of crime. However, the statistics given below may appear to be out of date, with a number of sources being around ten years old. While the following statistics provide a brief flavour of the numbers of those with a learning disability who may come to the attention of the legal system, Marshall-Tate *et al.* (2019) argue that the prevalence of people with a learning disability in the criminal justice system is unclear but that the "expert consensus is that people who have learning disabilities are over-represented".

- Between 20 and 30% of offenders at any one time have a learning difficulty or learning disability (Jacobson and Talbot, 2009, p. 5), bearing in mind that learning difficulties (dyslexia and dyscalculia) and learning disabilities are not the same thing. The Prison Reform Trust (Talbot, 2012) puts this figure somewhat lower, at between 10 and 20%.
- Over 60% of children who offend have communication difficulties and, of this group, around half have poor or very poor communication skills (Talbot, 2012).
- Around a quarter of children who offend have an IQ of less than 70 (Talbot, 2012). An intelligence quotient (IQ) is a total score derived from a set of standardised tests or subtests designed to assess human intelligence, the measurement of which is now seen as controversial. Approximately two-thirds of the population scores are between IQ 85 and IQ 115. This is seen as 'normal' or 'average' IQ.
- 7% of adult prisoners have an IQ of less than 70 and a further 25% have an IQ of 70–79 (Talbot, 2012, 2018).
- Almost 6000 men, women and children with an IQ of less than 70 (those who have a learning disability) are incarcerated in UK prisons at any given time.
- Prison inmates who have a learning disability are vulnerable to threats to their physical and psychological wellbeing and are more likely to be subject to control and restraint techniques.
- People with a disability are significantly more likely to be victims of crime than those without a disability. This gap is largest amongst those aged 16–34, where 39% of people with a disability reported having been a victim of crime, compared to 28% of people without a disability. A person with a limiting disability is at significantly greater risk of suffering violence or theft than a non-disabled person (DWP, 2014; Victim Support, 2016). Disability hate crimes recorded by the police in England and Wales increased by 9% from 2019 to 2020 (Home Office, 2020).

- People with a disability are less likely than their non-disabled peers to think the criminal justice system (CJS) is fair. This gap is largest amongst those aged 16–34, where 54% of people with a disability think that the CJS is fair, compared to 66% of people who do not have a disability (DWP, 2014).
- Those who are victims of hate crimes continue to be failed by the police, with many police officers neither properly investigating disability hate crimes nor treating victims as credible witnesses, according to a report by Mencap (Mencap, 2010).

ACTIVITY 8.1

Carry out an internet search around current statistics of people with a learning disability who come into contact with the criminal justice system, be that as perpetrators of crime, victims of crime or witnesses to a crime. How do the statistics that you discover differ from those given above? What are the likely statistical trends for the future based on the two sets of statistics?

8.4 A journey through forensic services

The journeys through the criminal justice service for Yasmin, Victoria and Brian (the three people we very briefly met at the start of this chapter) are likely to be long and complex. Given the diversity of the issues that surround them, their respective journeys will be very different. Their stories are highlighted below. In the cases of Victoria and Brian, the pathways given in Kingdon (2009, p. 377 (Appendix 12:1)) have been followed. There appear to be no similar pathways for victims or witnesses of crimes.

SCENARIO 8.1: VICTORIA

After being arrested, Victoria is taken to her local police station where she is assessed by the forensic medical examiner and then interviewed in the presence of an 'appropriate adult' (the local police station will likely have a list of people who could act as an 'appropriate adult'). At the interview, the role of the 'appropriate adult' is to protect the rights of vulnerable adults and children / minors in what is likely to be a highly stressful and often frightening environment and to ensure that those being arrested and interviewed are treated fairly and humanely. After the interviewing officer has sought advice regarding the most appropriate way to deal with Victoria, and given that this is not the first time that Victoria has been in contact with the police due to her behaviour, she is charged with possession of a Class B drug rather than just cautioned. Victoria is released on bail before being ordered to appear before the magistrates' court. Throughout the entire process, Victoria is supported by both the forensic and community learning disability nursing teams to understand why she has been arrested, what her rights are, the legal processes, what has happened to her at the police station and what is likely to happen to her over the next few weeks prior to and after appearing at the magistrates' court. It is explained to Victoria that as this is not the first time that she has come to the attention of the local police due to her behaviour, it is felt that a police caution would not be effective or appropriate at this time.

The magistrate, having again sought advice from appropriate support agencies, bases his decision on the fact that Victoria does have a learning disability and that a custodial sentence would not provide any real benefit for Victoria or society. The magistrate decides instead to sentence Victoria to non-custodial community service along with ongoing input regarding her use of drugs and antisocial behaviour. To this end, Victoria is offered support and guidance by the forensic learning disability and mental health teams.

SCENARIO 8.2: BRIAN

Brian is arrested at his home address as a result of a formal complaint being made by the victim and her parents. Brian is taken to the local police station where he is assessed by a forensic medical examiner (often a local GP who is contracted to provide medical services such as assessments on people who have been arrested) and then cautioned and interviewed in the presence of an 'appropriate adult'. Although the nature of the offence is serious, it is decided that to release Brian on police bail prior to appearing before the magistrates' court is the appropriate action to take. However, due to the nature of the offence, it is felt that to issue Brian with a police caution would not be appropriate.

Although Brian has apologised for his behaviour and promised that it would never happen again, because of the severity of the offence and the age of the victim (being under the age of consent), the magistrate invokes Section 35 of the Mental Health Act 1983 which permits for the hospital detention of a person for assessment. During his time within a community-based low secure unit, Brian is further assessed and supported to understand why he has acted as he did and to realise that his behaviour was wrong. He is also made aware of the effects and consequences of his actions on himself and others, including the possibility and effects of being placed on the 'sex offenders' register'. After a period within the low secure unit, Brian is reassessed and, as it is considered that he no longer poses a threat to society, released with ongoing support and supervision by the community forensic and learning disability teams.

SCENARIO 8.3: YASMIN

Yasmin is different from Brian and Victoria as she is a victim of crime rather than its perpetrator. While there is an increasing amount of literature around forensic services and perpetrators of crime, there appears to be very little in the way of researched evidence and information on forensic services and victims of crime. This apparent lack of research, information and resultant lack of support services for victims of crime is likely to be compounded by police officers not being able to recognise when a victim (and perpetrator for that matter) has a learning disability (Halstead, 1996). The ability to read, write and hold a conversation may mask the real level of disability and while the police may be good at recognising moderate or severe learning disability, those with a borderline or mild learning disability may be missed and their needs neither recognised nor met.

How Yasmin is approached by the desk officer at the police station could have either a positive or negative effect on her. As the bullying, victimisation and aggression that Yasmin and her family have experienced have occurred over a three-year period it is unlikely that this is the first time that the assistance of the local police has been sought. Trust or distrust of the police and legal system balances on such assistance and experiences.

It is likely that Yasmin will be asked if she would like to be taken to the local A&E department to have any physical injuries assessed and treated. It would be good practice for Yasmin to be offered the services of an 'appropriate adult' or advocate who could accompany her to the hospital. Once she feels able to do so, a statement of what happened would be taken and the perpetrators, if identified, brought to the police station for questioning. If the perpetrators are themselves children or minors (under the age of 18) then they may be vulnerable in their own right and may need access to similar 'appropriate adult'/advocacy services. Yasmin must be offered ongoing access to 'victim support' services as a matter of course. Victim Support, while being neither a government agency nor part of the police, is a national charity that gives free and confidential help to victims of crime, witnesses, their family, friends and anyone else affected across England and Wales. Victim Support also speaks out as a national voice for victims and witnesses and campaigns for change (www.victimsupport.org.uk).

8.5 The role of the nurse

We have already met Jill and Hanif from *Chapter 1*. Jill is a healthcare assistant who works in a GP practice and Hanif is a student nurse (adult branch) who is now completing a short assignment in a local police station as part of his learning disability placement. What are their roles in meeting the holistic needs of Victoria, Brian and Yasmin?

SCENARIO 8.1: VICTORIA AND SCENARIO 8.2: BRIAN

Hanif may well participate in the following:

- Observing and offering appropriate and supervised assistance in the physical, emotional and psychological assessment of Brian and Victoria
- Engaging in conversations with Brian and Victoria; this will, in part, gain their trust and could form part of the holistic assessment process
- Acting as an 'appropriate adult' if asked to do so during police interviews
- Advocating on behalf of Brian and Victoria whilst they are in custody
- Accompanying Brian and Victoria to the magistrates' court for moral support – it is unlikely that Hanif will have the necessary skills and knowledge to act as an 'expert witness' on behalf of either Brian or Victoria, this being the role of the forensic nursing team
- Visiting and supporting Brian in the low secure unit and Victoria during her community service and observing and participating in any rehabilitation programmes that Brian and Victoria will undergo.

Jill, the HCA, may be involved in the ongoing support through the provision of health checks of Brian and Victoria once they have been released or discharged back into the community. Jill may also be involved in the finding and securing of appropriate overnight or weekend respite care for Victoria so that her parents can have a break. Again, Jill may become involved in facilitating support groups not only for Victoria's parents and any siblings but also for other parents and siblings in a similar position. Finally, Jill may be involved in supporting Victoria's parents to obtain carers' benefit, carers' grants and access to local authority, NHS or voluntary sector-run carers' support services.

SCENARIO 8.3: YASMIN

Here, Hanif's role is likely to include:

- observing and offering appropriate assistance in the physical, emotional and psychological assessment of Yasmin
- engaging in conversations with Yasmin to gain her trust
- acting as an 'appropriate adult' and advocate during police interviews, and
- accompanying Yasmin to the local A&E so that she could have her injuries assessed and treated.

Again, as a placement project, Hanif could investigate the existence and effect of hate crimes against those with a learning disability within the community and of discrimination against those with disabilities within the healthcare systems.

It would be inappropriate for either Hanif or Jill to offer 'quick fix' approaches to long-standing disability hate crime such as that experienced by Yasmin and her family. Even the police appear to downplay the existence and effects of hate crimes on people with a learning disability and their families. It would certainly be inappropriate to suggest that Yasmin and her family move to a different area of town or a different town entirely, although on the surface such a move may result in a cessation of the hate crimes that they have experienced. Having said that, both Hanif and Jill could be aware of and involved in the Mencap campaign on hate crime (see Mencap's 'Hear my voice' campaign: www.mencap.org.uk/get-involved/campaign-mencap/hear-my-voice).

8.6 Conclusion

As can be seen, those with a learning disability are just as likely to come into contact with the various aspects of forensic services, whether that be as perpetrators, witnesses or victims of crime. These services and the issues and behaviour that are connected to forensic services tend to be complex and do not lend themselves to simple 'quick fix' solutions. Nonetheless, the roles of the forensic psychiatric team can be fascinating and rewarding areas to investigate further and to work in, as can the prison health services. Indeed, some healthcare assistants, nursing students and newly registered nurses and nursing associates may already be working in these fields. Riding, Swann and Swann (2005) may prove to be a useful resource for those who are in or considering such a role.

CHAPTER SUMMARY

Key points to take away from *Chapter 8*:
- ☑ Those with a learning disability are as likely as anyone else to come into contact with forensic services, be that as a witness, victim or perpetrator of a crime.
- ☑ Forensic services include the criminal justice system and a sub-branch of psychiatry that serves as the interface between the law, the various aspects of the criminal justice system, and psychiatry and residential or community mental health services.
- ☑ The role of the nurse will include reassuring the service user, offering psychological, emotional and practical support and acting as an 'appropriate adult' and advocate.

Questions

Question 8.1	What does forensic services mean in relation to those with a learning disability, and what comprises such services?
Question 8.2	What are the main differences in forensic care services as experienced by those who *engage in* as opposed to those who are *victims of* criminal activity?
Question 8.3	How many people with a learning disability live within your area? How many of these are likely to come into contact with forensic services either as 'perpetrators' or 'victims' of criminal activity and why?
Question 8.4	What are the roles of the nurse in supporting those who *engage in* criminal activity once they have been arrested?
Question 8.5	How do these roles differ to the roles indicated in supporting *victims of* criminal activity such as a hate crime?

REFERENCES

Barber, C. (2011) Support for learning disabilities in forensic services. *British Journal of Healthcare Assistants*, **5(10)**: 491–4.

Baxter, V. (2002) Nurses' perception of their role and skills in a medium secure unit. *Mental Health Nursing*, **11(30)**: 1312–19.

Burrow, S. (1993) An outline of the forensic nursing role. *British Journal of Nursing*, **2(18)**: 21–38.

Chaloner, C. and Coffey, M. (eds) (2000) *Forensic Mental Health Nursing: current approaches*. Blackwell Science.

Department for Work and Pensions (2014) *Disability facts and figures*. Available at: www.gov.uk/government/statistics/disability-facts-and-figures/disability-facts-and-figures (accessed 3 January 2022).

Halstead, S. (1996) Forensic psychiatry for people with a learning disability. *Advances in Psychiatric Treatment*, **2**: 76–85.

Home Office (2020) *Hate crime, England and Wales, 2019 to 2020*. Available at: www.gov.uk/government/statistics/hate-crime-england-and-wales-2019-to-2020/hate-crime-england-and-wales-2019-to-2020 (accessed 3 January 2022).

Jacobson, J. and Talbot, J. (2009) *Vulnerable Defendants in the Criminal Courts: a review of provision for adults and children*. Prison Reform Trust.

Kearns, A. (2001) Forensic services and people with learning disability: in the shadow of the Reed Report. *Journal of Forensic Psychiatry*, **12(1)**: 8–12.

Kettles, A., Peternelj-Taylor, C., Woods, P. *et al.* (2001) Forensic nursing: a global perspective. *British Journal of Forensic Practice*, **3(2)**: 29–41.

Kingdon, A. (2009) 'Forensic learning disability practice'. In Jukes, M. (ed.) *Learning Disability Nursing Practice*. Quay Books.

Marshall-Tate, K., Chaplin, E., Ali, S. and Hardy, S. (2019) Learning disabilities: supporting people in the criminal justice system. *Nursing Times* (online), **115(7)**: 22–6.

Mencap (2010) *Don't stand by: Hate crime research report*. Available at: www.mencap.org.uk/sites/default/files/2016-08/Don%27t%20stand%20by-research-report%20%281%29.pdf (accessed 3 January 2022).

Riding, T., Swann, C. and Swann, B. (eds) (2005) *The Handbook of Forensic Learning Disabilities*. Radcliffe Medical Press.

Royal College of Nursing (2019) *Nursing roles in forensic and justice services*. Available at: www.rcn.org.uk/clinical-topics/criminal-justice-services/nursing-roles-in-criminal-justice-services (accessed 3 January 2022).

Talbot, J. (2012) *Fair Access to Justice? Support for vulnerable defendants in the criminal courts*. Prison Reform Trust.

Talbot, J. (2018) *People with learning disabilities in prison*. Prison Reform Trust. Available at: www.rcpsych.ac.uk/docs/default-source/improving-care/ccqi/quality-networks/prison-quality-network-prison/past-pqn-events/pqn-15-march-2018/prisons-people-with-learning-disabilities-jenny-talbot.pdf (accessed 3 January 2022).

University of Central Lancashire (1999) *Nursing in Secure Environments*. UKCC.

Victim Support (2016) *Disabled people at increased risk of violent crime*. Available at: www.victimsupport.org.uk/press-releases/disabled-people-increased-risk-violent-crime-victim-support-research/ (accessed 3 January 2022).

FURTHER READING

Royal College of Nursing (RCN): Nursing in Justice and Forensic Health Care Forum: www.rcn.org.uk/get-involved/forums/nursing-in-justice-and-forensic-health-care-forum (accessed 3 January 2022).

Victim support: www.victimsupport.org.uk (accessed 3 January 2022).

Chapter 9
Sexuality and people with a learning disability

AIMS AND LEARNING OUTCOMES

The aims of this chapter are to:

- Highlight the meaning of sexuality

- Briefly highlight a variety of issues around sexuality and those with a learning disability

- Briefly discuss the law relating to sexual relationships and those with a learning disability

- Briefly discuss issues around consent to sexual activity

- Highlight the roles of the nurse in relation to the sexuality of those with a learning disability.

By the end of this chapter, you will be able to discuss:

- The meaning of sexuality and sex

- How the various aspects of human sexuality impact upon those with a learning disability

- The law and sexuality

- Issues around consent and sex

- Your role as a nurse or healthcare professional in promoting appropriate sexual health.

9.1 Introduction

Human sexuality, along with dying, death and bereavement, is perhaps one of the most difficult aspects of working with those who have a learning disability that nurses and health and social care professionals are likely to encounter. After all, sex and dying / death / bereavement are still very much socially taboo subjects; they are not common subjects for discussion with your mates at your local pub. They are the rather large 'elephants in the room'; they exist but few people even acknowledge them, let alone discuss them! Most people will just dance around the issues that are raised by human sexuality, often employing euphemisms in order to hide embarrassment. This could also apply to nurses. Therefore, within 'polite society', human sexuality and learning disability are likely to make for a very odd couple indeed!

However, to deny that those with a learning disability are sexual beings, that they have a right to their sexuality and that they have a right to experience and express their sexuality on the same basis as anyone else, is a gross denial of their human dignity, their human rights and of what, in part, makes them human.

9.2 What is sexuality?

Those with a learning disability are sexual beings, the same as me and you, and they have the same need and drive to sexually define, experience and express themselves as such. However, what is sexuality?

Sexuality could mean different things to different people at different times and in different cultures, with issues around self-identity, image, sensuality and sex being perhaps some of the more common and important concepts. Human sexuality focuses on a wide array of attributes and social activities and an abundance of behaviours, series of actions and societal attitudes. Again, sexuality can be seen as the quality or state of being sexual. Quite often, sexuality is an aspect of one's need for closeness, caring and touch. Generally speaking, human sexuality is how people experience and express themselves as sexual beings. Human sexuality also involves the capacity to have erotic experiences and responses.

Human sexuality may also involve a person's sexual attraction to another person which may be determined by their sexual orientation (gay, lesbian, bisexual or heterosexual ('straight')). Human sexuality impacts upon cultural, political, legal and philosophical aspects of life. It can refer to issues of morality, ethics, theology, spirituality or religion.

Within a wide variety of societies, sexuality can be defined, in part, by an increasing number of cultural contexts and governed by implied rules and social norms. Even within a single society (such as 'British', 'French', 'German' or 'Italian'), there are a number of often distinct and competing sub-cultures. By this it is meant that language, history and popular culture have roles to play in defining and promoting sexuality. One has only to see how colour mediates gender and sexuality in babies and very young children; even now, many baby girls are dressed in pink and baby boys in blue. As one gets older, more and more aspects of contemporary life and culture help to define, shape, present and express sexuality. Clothing colour, toys, play and social activities, music, TV programmes, films, sports, advertising and cosmetics are all examples of the culture of sexuality. However, as these are likely to be social and historical constructs, i.e. sexual meanings and norms that are 'artificially constructed' by society and social movements, such as the rise of feminism and the sexual revolution (Foucault, 1976), the experience and expression of sexuality can and quite often do change over time. Here time is seen in terms of decades and centuries on one level, and over the course of an individual's lifespan on another.

The age and manner in which children are informed of issues of sexuality are often hotly debated and are usually seen as a matter for parents and school-based sex education to resolve. Different countries hold varying views on when (ranging from age-appropriate preschool to puberty and teenage years) and how such sex education is presented, the contents of such education programmes and who teaches or presents these programmes. However, even within a single country, there are likely to be multiple and diverse cultures and therefore much discussion and conflict as to the nature, form and place of sex education programmes within that country.

9.3 Issues regarding sexuality and those with a learning disability

PAUSE FOR THOUGHT 9.1

Imagine if your sexuality was denied, decided or defined for you, or deemed to be wrong just because it exists. Hormones are not aware that they are seen by some as 'inappropriate' just because the bodies they inhabit are disabled. (Clark, 2014)

Sexuality is likely to encompass a wide range of relationships, behaviours and issues. This is true for everybody, whether they have a learning disability or not. Some of these issues will include many of the following:

- Gender issues: the complex interplay of historical and current social and cultural influences and expectations that help to shape a person's sexual identity
- Puberty: a developmental and maturation stage which marks the start of the transition between childhood and adulthood that everyone experiences, whether or not they have a learning disability; Wrobel (2003), Hartman (2014) and Asayba, Burns and Doswell (2019) provide a wealth of useful information that could be invaluable when supporting pre-teenagers or teenagers with a learning disability and their parents
- Masturbation: if done in private, this is a normal means of sexual release
- Sexual relationships
- Contraception
- Marriage
- Pregnancy, either within or outside marriage
- Same-sex relationships
- Alternative forms of sexual expression such as receiving and giving physical pain for sexual pleasure, bondage and fetish wear and pornography (both 'straight' and 'gay / lesbian').

Those with a learning disability are people first and learning disabled second. Thus, those with a learning disability have the same rights and drives as anyone else to engage in sexual activities, and having a learning disability must not preclude engagement in such activities. However, those with a learning disability also have a right to protection from the negative consequences of such sexual activities, such as sexually transmitted infections (STIs), and advice must be sought from the multidisciplinary team if it is believed that a person or couple with a learning disability is sexually active and at risk of contracting an STI.

People with profound and multiple learning disabilities (PMLD) such as Thomas, who we met in *Chapter 3*, are likely to have the same needs and rights to explore their bodies, to derive pleasure from doing so and to express and experience their sexuality, as anyone else. However, as a result of the profound level of their learning disability they would be unable to validly give, withhold or withdraw voluntary consent to any form of sexual relationship (Mencap, undated (a)). Therefore, it would be illegal for anyone to engage in a sexual relationship with those with a PMLD. Having said that, the sexuality of those with a PMLD, as for other people with a learning disability, can be asserted through the use of clothing fashions, hair styles, cosmetics, room décor and 'gender-biased' music styles and social activities.

However, those with a learning disability can be both victims and perpetrators of sexual abuse. Sexual abuse or abusive relationships occur when consent to such sexual or emotional / 'romantic' relationships or activities was not freely given by either party. This could involve a range of behaviours ranging from unwanted sexual attention, nuisance phone calls, 'sexting' (the sending of text messages with a sexual content) and stalking, to sexual assault and rape. Forced marriages and female genital mutilation, both prevalent in certain cultures, are also forms of sexual abuse. Again, the administration of oral contraception without the person's knowledge or consent and the administration of certain hormones to either slow down or prevent the onset of puberty (particularly in females) (both of which occurred during the 1960s through to the 1980s) can be seen to be abusive. Some of these issues and behaviours could arise from a lack of knowledge, awareness and understanding of what comprises appropriate sexual behaviour and ways of responding to such behaviour and could be addressed through education.

9.4 **The law**

Those with a learning disability are both subject to and protected by the same legislation that every other person is subject to and protected by. Within the UK, no one under the age of 16 can consent legally to sex regardless of ability (although this age of consent may differ in other countries) and sex with a child under 12 years of age is considered to be statutory rape. According to the Sexual Offences Act 2003 it is an offence to engage in "sexual activity with a person with a mental disorder impeding choice". A person with a serious or profound learning disability, by the nature of this definition, is unlikely to have the capacity to consent to sexual activity (i.e. to understand what it means and its possible consequences). This means they are likely to fall into the category of a person who has a 'mental disorder impeding choice'. However, as this is a grey area for those with a borderline and mild learning disability, it may not apply to the same degree given that such people are likely to be more aware of choices and their consequences and thus more likely to be able to consent.

It is also an offence to:

- cause or incite a person with a mental disorder impeding choice to engage in sexual activity
- engage in sexual activity in the presence of a person with a mental disorder impeding choice
- cause a person with a mental disorder impeding choice to watch a sexual act.

Although intended to act as safeguards for those who are likely to be vulnerable to sexual abuse and exploitation because of their learning disability, the problem here is that this could potentially become a blanket ban on all legitimate sexual expression, experience and activity on the part of those with a learning disability. Therefore, great care must be taken to ensure that those with a learning disability are protected from sexual, physical, mental and emotional harm through sexual exploitation, whilst acknowledging that they are sexual beings and have the same right as anyone else to express and experience their sexuality. For more information see Mencap (undated (a)).

9.5 Issues around consent

It could be suggested that consent and the ability to give consent are the central issues that need to be considered in relation to sex and people with a learning disability. It must be remembered here that any sexual act such as intimate touching or kissing without consent is sexual assault and that having sex with a person without that person's consent is rape. It must also be remembered that consent to kissing or the holding of hands is not the same as, nor does it imply, consent by the person to having sex. This applies to everyone, regardless of whether or not that person has a learning disability.

In England and Wales, the relevant legislation is in the Sexual Offences Act 2003 and the Mental Capacity Act 2005 (Thompson, 2011). For people aged 16 and over, section 74 of the Sexual Offences Act says: "A person consents if he or she agrees by choice and has the freedom and capacity to make that choice". Without such consent, an offence has been committed. It is also illegal for staff and volunteers to have sex with the people they support and care for (Thompson, 2011).

The Mental Capacity Act 2005 formed the central component of *Chapter 6*, where the meanings of mental capacity and consent and how to assess a person's ability or mental capacity to give a valid consent were discussed. Put simply, consent, which could either be explicit or implicit and verbal, written or gestural, refers to the provision of approval or agreement between two or more people or between a person and an organisation, particularly and especially after thoughtful consideration, for an action to take place. For the purposes of Section 2 of the Act, a person is unable to make a decision for himself if he is unable to: understand the information relevant to the decision, retain that information, use or weigh that information as part of the process of making the decision and communicate his decision (whether by talking, using sign language or any other means).

There are a number of principles within the Mental Capacity Act 2005 that may be relevant to assessing whether a person with a learning disability has the necessary mental capacity to consent to a sexual relationship. These include:

- Assume capacity: many people with learning disabilities are likely to have the mental capacity to engage in sex and relationships.
- Support people to make their own decisions: provide appropriate and accessible information on relationships, healthy living and sex education.
- People can make unwise choices: a bad relationship is a mistake we can all make.
- If someone lacks capacity, the decision must be in their best interests: assess capacity to consent to sex.
- Try to limit restrictions on the person's rights and freedom: where an individual lacks capacity to consent to sex it may not always be in their best interests to stop opportunities for sexual contact.

In order for consent to be valid, those with a learning disability should understand what sex involves physically and emotionally, and that it should feel good. They should also understand the potential consequences of sex, such as pregnancy, STIs and the risk of emotional hurt, as well as the importance of consent for both parties involved, including the right to say no (Thompson, 2011). However, Thompson also suggests that the most difficult capacity assessments involve people with learning disabilities who agree to have sex but may lack insight into the other person's motives. Examples may include the woman with a learning disability agreeing to have sex on the promise of a relationship, but not understanding that the man is only interested in sex, or a man with a learning disability thinking he has a girlfriend, but she is mainly interested in his benefits or having somewhere free to stay. In either of these scenarios, the person with a learning disability may be the victim of a crime under the Sexual Offences Act 2003.

It is likely that there may be a number of people with a learning disability who are gay, lesbian or bisexual. However, those who are face enormous challenges to 'come out' as such, and it may be some time before significant numbers are able to make this choice for themselves (Abbott and Howarth, 2005; Clark, 2014; Mencap, undated (b)).

It should be borne in mind that mental capacity assessments can be subjective, and two different care professionals may come to different conclusions about the same case. If a consensus cannot be achieved, it may be necessary to ask the Court of Protection to decide on a person's mental capacity to consent to engaging in a sexual relationship.

9.6 The role of the nurse

Jill (briefly introduced in *Chapter 1*) is a healthcare assistant who works in a GP practice three days a week and a local community health centre for the remaining two days. In both settings, she works with a number of people ranging from 15 to 70 years of age who have a learning disability. Jill is interested in providing effective support to her patients/service users in the area of sexual health.

Human sexuality involves many complex emotional, ethical, social, cultural, moral and legal issues. Simplistic responses to the questions and queries being posed by her service users, their families and healthcare colleagues, are likely to be unhelpful, inappropriate and bordering on the unprofessional. However, there are a number of things that Jill can do in order to provide an effective support service.

- Although she is a healthcare assistant and not a registered nurse and as such is not (yet) subject to the professional code of conduct for nurses, it would be good practice for Jill to be aware of, understand and work within the Nursing and Midwifery Council's (NMC) code of professional conduct. She must never forget that she is personally and professionally accountable for her actions (or lack of them).

- Jill needs to be aware of, understand and implement fully any employer and organisational procedures, policies and guidelines around the issues of sexuality, sexual health and consent, regardless of who the service user or patient is.

- Jill needs to be aware of and understand that she does not work in a social, ethical, philosophical or cultural vacuum. Therefore, she must be aware of and understand social and professional attitudes and beliefs regarding sexuality, many of which may be found within herself or her colleagues and how these issues, attitudes and beliefs impact upon what she does and how she does it.

- Jill must actively listen in a compassionate and non-judgemental manner that considers both what the service users are saying and what they are not saying in terms of their sexuality and how they perceive and experience that sexuality.

- Jill could ensure, within the bounds of accepted good practice, training in sexuality, organisational policies and professional codes of conduct, that accurate and up-to-date information regarding a wide range of sexual issues such as puberty, contraception, STIs, straight or same-sex relationships, alternative sexual expressions such as fetishism, BDSM, pregnancy and childbirth and parenthood are made available in a variety of formats including online / downloadable videos or other visual formats (for laptops and smartphones), easy read and visual (line drawings, pictures and photos). Just because a person has a learning disability does not mean that they should be denied the opportunity to explore, experience and express their sexuality in their own way, as long as such sexual expression is consensual.

- There are a number of healthcare resources that Jill could access for advice and support in order to assist her service users. These could include hospital-based learning disability liaison nurses, the local learning disability services or mainstream sexual healthcare or health promotion professionals.

- Likewise, there is an increasing range of external support agencies that Jill may find useful in terms of information, advice and contact. These support agencies, such as BILD, Mencap, the Down's Syndrome Association and the National Autistic Society, produce information leaflets on sexuality in all its forms and expressions, safer sex, relationships and healthy living that are targeted at people with a learning disability (often in an 'easy read' format) or care professionals and can be located and downloaded, often free of charge, from their respective websites. TV programmes such as *The Undateables*, a British TV documentary series that follows a range of people on dates who have long-term conditions, including learning and other disabilities, and developmental disorders, may also be useful in terms of information. The series works in conjunction with the dating agency, Flame Introductions, and was broadcast on Channel 4.

■ Again, small organisations, often set up and run by those with disabilities, may also be useful sources of information. Included in the latter would be Outsiders (https://outsiders.org.uk). Outsiders is both an online peer support and 'real world' social club specifically run by and for those with a range of disabilities. Outsiders is a place where a person and their sexuality will be accepted and their personal problems addressed. Social events often revolve around shared meals.

■ Jill could also seek the advice of the sexuality support team where such teams exist (see box below) before implementing any sexual health programmes. The CQC publication *Relationships and sexuality in adult social care services* (www.cqc. org.uk/sites/default/files/20190221-Relationships-and-sexuality-in-social-care-PUBLICATION.pdf) may prove useful as a resource to assist Jill.

■ Jill could set up and sensitively facilitate focus groups comprising those with a learning disability to explore the thoughts, feelings, knowledge levels and person-centred needs around sexuality. The findings of such focus groups could then lead to:

■ Jill setting up and sensitively facilitating workshops on sexuality, healthy living and lifestyles, personal safety and parenting (Brickley, 2003; Woodhouse, Green and Davies, 2001). Such workshops could include many of the issues covered briefly in the sections above. To avoid the problems that could arise through a perception on the part of service users that Jill is 'preaching' a healthy lifestyle message, such workshop sessions must be run by those with a learning disability and be guided by their wants, needs and agenda.

What is a Sexuality Support Team?

The Sexuality Support Team, run by the Hertfordshire Partnership University NHS Foundation Trust (SST, formerly Consent) offered a range of services to respond to a broad range of sexuality issues affecting women and men with learning disabilities, including enabling informed choices, sexual health, issues of HIV risks, and working with people with learning disabilities who have been sexually abused or perpetrated sexual abuse.

The team had a multidisciplinary approach and had a national profile for quality and experience. The SST was part of Hertfordshire Partnership NHS Trust, but offered its services across the UK and aimed to work in partnership with other individuals and organisations. Services included consultancy, group work, training, individual work, workshops, conferences and student placements.

As other NHS Trusts may operate something similar to this, it may be helpful to contact the local hospital-based learning disability liaison nurse or community learning disability services for advice, suggestions or support.

Contact the local hospital-based learning disability liaison nurse, the local learning disability community team, Mencap or BILD regarding the existence of a sexuality support team (SST) in your area. If there is no SST in your area (and it is likely that there will not be), seek advice and guidance regarding sexuality from the local learning disability liaison nurse and reflect upon the need for such a service, considering the possibility of establishing such a service as a post-registration project.

9.7 Conclusion

As those with a learning disability develop and grow older, their sexuality is a fact of life which needs to be faced, accepted and engaged with. Those who work with people who have a learning disability walk a very thin tightrope when it comes to those people's sexuality. On the one hand, nurses, nursing students and HCAs have a professional and common-law duty of care and protection to those who have a learning disability (just as they have to any other vulnerable patient or service user). On the other hand, those with a learning disability have a basic human right to experience, express and enjoy their sexuality on the same basis as anyone else. This right must be remembered and acted upon appropriately at all times.

CHAPTER SUMMARY

Key points to take away from *Chapter 9*:
- ☑ Those with a learning disability have the same sexual needs, desires and drives as anyone else in society.
- ☑ Sexuality means different things to different people at different times and in different cultures, with issues around self-identity, image, sensuality and sex being perhaps some of the more common and important concepts.
- ☑ Sexuality can be asserted through the use of clothing fashions, hair styles, cosmetics, room décor and 'gender-biased' music styles and social activities.
- ☑ The Sexual Offences Act 2003 put in place a range of measures to safeguard those with a learning disability from sexual abuse.
- ☑ Consent and the ability to give consent is the central issue that needs to be considered in relation to sex and people with a learning disability.

Questions

Question 9.1	What does sexuality mean to you?
Question 9.2	What is the law regarding sex and those with a learning disability?
Question 9.3	What are the issues that people with a learning disability experience regarding their sexuality?
Question 9.4	How would having a learning disability affect some people's ability to consent to engage in sexual relationships or activity?
Question 9.5	How would you safeguard a person's right to engage in sexual relationships and activities?
Question 9.6	How would you safeguard a person with a learning disability from potential harm?

REFERENCES

Abbott, D. and Howarth, J. (2005) *Secret Loves, Hidden Lives?: exploring issues for people with learning difficulties who are gay, lesbian or bisexual.* Policy Press.

Asagba, K., Burns, J. and Doswell, J. (2019) *Sex and Relationships Education for Young People and Adults with Intellectual Disabilities and Autism.* Pavilion Publishing.

Brickley, S. (2003) 'Working with parents who have a learning disability and their children'. In Jukes, M. and Bollard, M. (eds) (2003) *Contemporary Learning Disability Practice.* Quay Books.

Clark, N. (2014) *Let's talk about sex.* Enable. Available at: http://enablemagazine.co.uk/nicky-clark-lets-talk-about-sex/ (accessed 3 January 2022).

Foucault, M. (1976) *The History of Sexuality Vol. 1: an introduction.* Editions Gallimard.

Hartman, D. (2014) *Sexuality and Relationship Education for Children and Adolescents with Autism Spectrum Disorders: a professional's guide*. Jessica Kingsley Publishers.

Mencap (undated (a)) *Sexuality and relationships – FAQs*. Available at: www.mencap.org.uk/advice-and-support/relationships-and-sex/sexuality-and-relationships-faqs (accessed 3 January 2022).

Mencap (undated (b)) *Sexuality – research and statistics*. Available at: www.mencap.org.uk/learning-disability-explained/research-and-statistics/sexuality-research-and-statistics (accessed 3 January 2022).

Thompson, D. (2011) Decisions about sex for people with learning disabilities. *Nursing Times*, **107** (online).

Woodhouse, A., Green, G. and Davies, S. (2001) Parents with learning disabilities: service audit and development. *British Journal of Learning Disabilities*, **29**: 128–132.

Wrobel, M. (2003) *Taking Care of Myself: a hygiene, puberty and personal curriculum for young people with autism*. Future Horizons.

RESOURCE

Mencap (2019) *Sexuality and relationships resources*. Available at: www.mencap.org.uk/sites/default/files/2019-10/Sexuality%20and%20Relationships%20Resources%20Mencap%202019_0.pdf (accessed 3 January 2022).

Chapter 10
Ageing and those with a learning disability

AIMS AND LEARNING OUTCOMES

The aims of this chapter are to:

- Discuss the meaning of old age
- Highlight normal ageing
- Highlight a number of medical, physiological, neurological and sensory issues associated with the ageing process
- Highlight issues around dementia
- Briefly highlight the role of the nurse.

By the end of this chapter, you will be aware of, understand and be able to discuss:

- The meaning of old age
- What constitutes 'normal ageing'
- The impact of a number of medical issues associated with ageing
- The impact of dementia on those with a learning disability
- Existing support structures and services for those with a learning disability
- The need for both generic and specific services for those with a learning disability
- Your role as a nurse, a nursing student or an HCA
- In addition to these, you will be able to begin implementing some of the ideas that can be found in this chapter.

SCENARIO 10.1: JIM

Jim, a 67-year-old gentleman with a severe learning disability, is experiencing the early stages of Alzheimer's dementia. Jim lives in a residential home for those with a learning disability along with four other people, where the average age of the residents is 60 and the youngest resident is 50.

10.1 Introduction

Life expectancy for those with a learning disability has been slowly increasing since the 1920s, to the point where many of those with a learning disability are now expected to live into what would normally be seen as 'old age' (Down's Syndrome Association, 2018a; NICE, 2018). Yet those with a learning disability will still die significantly younger than those without a learning disability (NHS Digital, 2020). However, it has only been fairly recently that any serious thought has been given to the possibility that those with a learning disability may reach and live well into old age, a situation that is compounded by a lack of information on appropriate elderly care. Consequently, whilst services and resources for those who are elderly and do not have a learning disability exist and are usually excellent, the existence of both generic and specific care and support services for people who have a learning disability as they enter and live through old age may range from non-existent to excellent via poor, patchy and good.

As a nurse working in a general hospital, GP practice, health centre, community nursing team or elderly residential care services, you are likely to meet and work with people with a learning disability who are experiencing old age.

10.2 What is old age?

PAUSE FOR THOUGHT 10.1

When does old age occur? Does one actually know when one reaches old age? Does it matter?

The inclusion of the two poems (*Warning* and *Radio 2*) referred to below, although light-hearted, is intended to question attitudes related to ageing and what is considered to be 'appropriate old age-related behaviour'.

PAUSE FOR THOUGHT 10.2: HUMOROUS POEMS ON AGEING

Is ageing and old age a state of mind? Before reading the remainder of this chapter, read the two humorous poems on ageing (the first of these two may be familiar to many of you):

- *Warning* by Jenny Joseph (available at: www.poemhunter.com/poem/warning/) (about a woman's rebellion against ageing)
- *Radio 2* by Dean Farnell (available at: www.dennydavis.net/poemfiles/aging2b.htm).

For some of us, old age is so far away that it does not even register; for others, it is just around the corner beckoning to us! Yet, do we actually know what old age is and when middle age ends and old age starts? Is a basic meaning of old age applicable to everyone?

It could be suggested that old age is very much a 'moveable feast', with those who have reached the retirement age of 66 considering themselves or being considered to be moving into old age. Yet, many people who are in their 70s and beyond still consider themselves to be 'middle-aged' or youthful, at least in spirit! One has only to look at the main characters in the television sitcom *Last of the Summer Wine* that can still be viewed on YouTube and certain digital TV channels! Is there a mismatch between what a person's body is telling them and what their mind and soul are telling them? This debate is pertinent when one considers that many people who are in their 70s are still working for a living, some in very high profile and very demanding roles – Pope Francis, for example, was 76 when he took office in March 2013 and Joe Biden was 78 when he was elected US President!

Again, those with a learning disability are known to have a life expectancy below that of those without a learning disability (NHS Digital, 2020). However, they also tend to experience many of the health issues that are associated with old age, such as dementia, well before their 'non-disabled' peers.

For the sake of expediency, the current retirement age of 66 will be taken as marking the end of middle age and the start of old age. However, as the age of retirement will rise to 68 for those born in or after the 1990s, so should the start of 'old age'.

10.3 Normal ageing

As can be seen from the two poems cited above, ageing can be rather bittersweet, with a gradual rather than abrupt onset. Physical appearance may change: grey hair to be replaced by white hair and smooth skin by wrinkles. Many will remember with clarity and perhaps with some sadness their youth and may try to deny their advancing years. I, for example, fully intend to enter my 70s and 80s still listening to and enjoying Pink Floyd, Gong and Genesis (the Peter Gabriel years of course)! There are likely to be grandchildren and even great-grandchildren to enjoy and embarrass. The mortgage will be paid off and there may be more money and time for leisure activities such as the University of the Third Age (U3A), travel, gardening, and arts and crafts. Meeting friends for tea, coffee or the odd pint or two may become more important as methods of social engagement. The need for personal reflection on one's life, the need for reconciliation with friends and family members and personal religious faith, beliefs and activity may become more important during the ageing process.

More negative aspects of normal ageing include the realisation of one's own mortality and having a finite time left to live. More and more of one's friends and family will die (although only in my sixties, I am aware of around half a dozen people from my own year at secondary school who have died). The body may start to show major signs of 'wear and tear' and consequently many people who are elderly may need greater assistance with normal activities of daily living. There may be more social isolation, loneliness and consequent depression.

10.4 Common medical conditions

Although those with a learning disability who are elderly are at vastly increased risk of developing dementia (Down's Syndrome Association, 2018b), there is a wide range of health and physical conditions which they are also at increased risk of developing. However, these may not be recognised as such, because nurses may feel that these conditions are part of the person's learning disability rather than the effects of ageing. These health and social conditions are likely to include some or many of the following:

Visual impairment. Ouldred and Bryant (2008) suggest that visual impairment, up to and including becoming registered blind, is likely to increase with age and level of disability and may even be higher in those with a learning disability. This is particularly marked in those with Down's syndrome (Wallace and Dalton, 2006). It appears that the most frequent form of visual impairment in those with a learning disability is cataracts, with a prevalence rate of around 40% in people with Down's syndrome (Kiani and Miller, 2010).

Hearing impairment. As with visual impairment, hearing impairment also increases with age and again is more common in those with learning disabilities, particularly Down's syndrome (Wallace and Dalton, 2006; Kiani and Miller, 2010; Down's Syndrome Association, 2018a).

Depression. Many elderly people are likely to experience depression for a variety of reasons, including social isolation, loneliness, the death of family and friends, the person's own impending death and increasing physical and sensory frailties. Given that those with a learning disability are more likely to experience depression (see *Chapter 7*), it is likely that those who have a learning disability will not only experience age-related depression but may do so more than those who do not have a learning disability.

Hypothyroidism. Hypothyroidism can occur in 20–30% of people with Down's syndrome (Ouldred and Bryant, 2008; Down's Syndrome Association, 2018a). This means that the thyroid gland does not produce enough hormones. Common signs of an underactive thyroid, some of which can mimic certain signs and symptoms of dementia, are tiredness, weight gain, functional decline and feeling depressed. An underactive thyroid is not usually serious and can often be treated successfully by taking daily hormone replacement tablets such as thyroxine.

Coronary artery disease. This is a disease of the arteries that supply blood to the heart and is the second most common cause of death amongst those with a learning disability; it is increasing as a result of the rise in life expectancy and lifestyle changes (Ouldred and Bryant, 2008; Down's Syndrome Association, 2018a). Up to 50% of those with Down's syndrome have some form of congenital heart defect which exposes those with such defects to increased risk of strokes and heart attacks.

Epilepsy. Drugs used to manage and treat epilepsy may cause drowsiness and problems with physical coordination and movement, both of which may be confused with dementia symptoms.

Diabetes. Although the prevalence of both type 1 and 2 diabetes in people with learning disabilities is unknown, it is generally thought (Ouldred and Bryant, 2008) that both types are more common than in those without a learning disability. However, Diabetes UK (2018) suggests that those with a learning disability are twice at risk of developing diabetes than those who do not have a learning disability. Complications associated with diabetes, including retinopathy, neuropathy and nephropathy, are likely to increase with age.

Arthritis and other musculoskeletal conditions. These are conditions that affect people increasingly as they get older and which negatively affect their physical mobility and dexterity, with pain becoming increasingly difficult to manage. This is true for both those with and without a learning disability, although the onset of arthritis in those with a learning disability could well be earlier (Down's Syndrome Association, 2018a). Thus, meeting their own personal hygiene needs, opening items such as bottles, cans or jars, using ordinary cutlery and getting out of the house become increasingly difficult.

Social isolation. Social isolation is not inevitable as a result of advancing age and its accompanying physical and health issues. However, as a result of increasing sensory, memory, physical and mobility difficulties, increasing numbers of elderly people appear to lose confidence in going out independently. This may result in a gradual decline in social contact and interaction and the loss of friends, some of whom may also be experiencing social isolation for similar reasons. Those with a learning disability may already experience such social isolation as a result of their existing disabilities and may thus feel any increased isolation more keenly.

10.5 **Dementia**

Ouldred and Bryant (2008, p. 89) suggest that "as people with pre-existing intellectual impairment grow older, they become subject to developing the same health conditions and problems as the older general population". This is confirmed by the Down's Syndrome Association (2018b). They also suggest that the prevalence of dementia is much higher in those with a learning disability and that many health and social care professionals are unaware of, or do not understand the increased risk of Alzheimer's dementia or its symptoms in people with learning disabilities. Indeed, Prasher (1995) suggests that dementia, the most prevalent form of which is Alzheimer's disease, can be present in around 36% of those with a learning disability who are aged 50–59. The Alzheimer's Society (undated) has suggested that one in 50 people with Down's syndrome develop dementia in their 30s, rising sharply to more than half of those who live to 60 or over. By comparison, the number of people among the population without a learning disability who are aged 60–69 and who develop dementia is about one in 75. Although deterioration in other human faculties such as mobility, sight and hearing can normally be seen within an elderly population, it is perhaps dementia that is most commonly identified with old age. This is also particularly true for those with a learning disability.

Ouldred and Bryant (2008, p. 90) suggest that dementia is a syndrome that affects memory, thinking, orientation, comprehension, calculation, learning capacity, language and judgement. Alzheimer's disease is characterised by a build-up of abnormal proteins between nerve cells and a reduction of chemical neurotransmitters such as acetylcholine. There is a gradual progression of the disease, starting from the area of the brain that controls and regulates short-term surface memory and which will eventually affect all areas of the brain.

10.5.1 Assessment of dementia

Early diagnosis of dementia conditions in people with a learning disability is likely to be complex. However, it is vital in order that conditions such as depression and thyroid problems, which may mimic some of the symptoms of dementia, can be treated and then ruled out. According to Ouldred and Bryant (2008), the best place to carry out a diagnostic assessment for dementia is in the person's own home, as this is likely to be the most familiar and non-threatening environment for the person.

There have been a number of studies into the diagnosis of dementia conditions in people with a learning disability. For example, DC–LD, the classification system developed by the Royal College of Psychiatrists (2001), is one of the tools that are often used to diagnose dementia, and Aylward *et al.* (1997) have published international guidelines on the diagnostic criteria for the diagnosis of dementia conditions in people with a learning disability. Dementia UK (2019) has also published useful information regarding dementia and those with a learning disability.

When assessing adults with a learning disability such as Jim (see *Scenario 10.1*) in order to diagnose possible dementia, the following may be useful:

- Jim's physical appearance and the appearance of his immediate environment
- Perceptions
- Jim's mood: does he appear depressed?
- Thought process
- Insight: is Jim aware of what is happening to him?
- Does Jim express and experience compulsive and repetitive rituals?
- Has Jim's personality changed?
- Is Jim oriented to person, time, place, memory or language? Does he know who and where he is and what day of the week, month of the year or year it is?

Much of the evidence for the above can be gained through spending time and interacting with Jim and observing him around the home where he lives. The home's care staff, other care professionals and Jim's care, nursing and medical notes will also be a valuable source of information. Such sources of information become even more important if Jim does not have or loses the ability to communicate verbally.

10.6 The role of the nurse

With advancing old age of those with a learning disability and its accompanying mental, sensory and physical frailty and possible isolation, the roles of the nurse are likely to be many, varied and challenging.

First of all, there is a need to understand the ageing process and its associated health conditions, such as dementia, and how this process can affect the person. This could be achieved through engaging in professional development opportunities such as workshops, short courses (some of which can be accessed online and therefore engaged in away from the everyday work environment and in one's own time) and the reading of journal articles around the ageing process and care for the elderly.

Secondly, try to resist the temptation of approaching and treating all those with a learning disability who are elderly together as one group. They are individuals first and foremost and then elderly learning disabled; they deserve and have the right to be treated accordingly! Having said that, there are a number of ideas and practices which those working with people who have a learning disability and are elderly could find useful, including:

- Verbal and gestural reassurance being given to those such as Jim who are experiencing age-related health conditions.
- Accurate and current information regarding the various healthcare issues being experienced by Jim must be made available to him in a format and manner, and at a time appropriate to his needs, levels of understanding and ways of communicating. It must be remembered that Jim's ability to consent to treatment and nursing care and interventions will be predicated on the availability and presentation of such information.
- Pharmaceutical management of some of the symptoms of dementia. Remember that there is no known cure for dementia. However, cholinesterase inhibitors appear to be effective in the symptomatic slowing down and relief of cognitive decline (Ouldred and Bryant, 2008).
- Reality orientation and validation, which aims to maintain and improve the person's orientation and awareness of their environment through a variety of prompts and activities (Ouldred and Bryant, 2008). Validation therapy focuses on the importance of an individual's feelings and their attempts to express them instead of correcting factual errors in communications. The true meanings behind the communication are sought.
- Reminiscence therapy seeks to encourage recollections and memories of details or events of an individual's life. Reminiscence therapy, which can take place either one-to-one or in a small group setting, can have a positive effect on a person's autobiographical memory, socialisation, long-term memory, communication and social interaction and engagement.
- Some, like Jim, will live in a local authority, health service or independent sector care home. The care home staff may need support in meeting Jim's holistic and person-centred care needs.

Again, resist the temptation to 'overshadow'. Diagnostic overshadowing occurs when a healthcare professional assumes that the behaviour of a person with learning disabilities is part of their disability without exploring other factors such as physical or biological issues. Overshadowing can be defined in the following way: "once a diagnosis is made of a major condition… there is a tendency to attribute all other problems to that diagnosis, thereby leaving other co-existing conditions undiagnosed" (Neurotrauma Law Nexus, undated). Thus, a change in Jim's behaviour may be attributed to his learning disability rather than due to pain as a result of arthritis, decrease in sensory ability or the onset of dementia, all of which can often be connected to the ageing process. Nurses can play a crucial role in reducing clinical risks inherent in diagnostic overshadowing whilst working with Jim, ensuring that health professionals see the person and not just his disability. Emerson and Baines (2010) have highlighted that when treating a person with a learning disability, "symptoms of physical ill-health are mistakenly attributed to either a mental health/behavioural problem or as being inherent in the person's learning disabilities."

ACTIVITY 10.1

List four ways in which overshadowing could affect those with a learning disability.

List four ways in which you could challenge these.

ACTIVITY 10.2

Choose any three of the sensory, physical, mental and social issues from the previous two sections. Devise a brief care assessment and care plan that would assist a 68-year-old person with a learning disability who is experiencing these issues.

The provision of domiciliary care and support for those who live on their own with multi-agency support could be invaluable not only in the meeting of physical needs such as dressing/undressing, nutrition/hydration, mobility and personal hygiene but in social communication, interaction and engagement. Remember that one of the major issues that many elderly people have to face on a daily basis is social isolation.

Likewise, specialist daily living equipment should be provided, such as magnifying glasses (to enable those with declining eyesight to read printed material such as letters, books and newspapers), bottle and can openers, raised toilet seats, large-handled cutlery and mobility aids such as walking frames. These can all be obtained through the local physiotherapy team, local disability equipment stockists (check online for details of these) or disability trade exhibitions such as Naidex (see its website: www.naidex.co.uk).

The support, information and resources that can be provided by the various voluntary organisations for those who are elderly should not be overlooked. Age UK, for example, has a very informative website that covers many of the issues experienced by those who are elderly (www.ageuk.org.uk). Age UK also runs local support groups, drop-in centres for those who are 'informal caregivers' and outreach services. Although not specifically targeted at those with a learning disability, much of the contents of the Age UK website is likely to be relevant.

When working with a person with dementia, a range of resources are available including:

- Dementia cafés, which are free to visit, offer a place to socialise over a cup of tea or coffee and biscuits, learn more about dementia and local services, and enjoy something new each session. They can be situated anywhere in the UK but are normally at a local day centre or local meeting place with easy access. There are many useful resources all under one roof with many people in a similar situation to the person with dementia and their families. Any subject that might help you to better deal with living with or caring for somebody who has a form of dementia can be discussed, and legal advice can often be offered. Dementia cafés are relatively easy and cheap to set up and run, as they only require a meeting space and basic refreshments and access to accessible information and dementia care specialists. Further information on dementia cafés can be found at: www.dementia.co.uk/support/dementia-cafe.
- Old-style grocery and sweet shops that accept 'pre-decimalisation' currency (pounds, shillings, sixpenny and thrupenny pieces, pennies, ha'pennies, farthings). Many nursing and care homes and day centres are beginning to see the value of these, not only as a social activity but as an aid to memory. Finding sweets, drinks and food that may not be available today but would have been available in the 1950s and 1960s may prove to be difficult and advice should be obtained from dementia organisations.
- Likewise, many nursing and care homes and day centres have sectioned off a corner of a lounge or 'day room' and turned it into a mini pub which acts as a social hub as well as promoting and preserving memory retention.

Given the additional intellectual / cognitive issues and needs of those with a learning disability, providing dementia cafés, 'pubs' and shops selling sweets and food items from the 1950s will need to be tailor-made to meet these additional needs. Those with a learning disability born in the 1940s would be very likely to have lived significant parts of their lives, possibly from their early infancy, in long-stay institutions and would thus not have had the same social experiences or opportunities as their 'non-learning disabled' peers.

It must also be remembered that an emphasis must be placed not only on the likely decline in sensory, physical and cognitive health and abilities often associated with old age, but on how to live well and enjoy one's post-retirement years. Re-read the two poems suggested at the start of this chapter and, if possible, watch an episode of *Last of the Summer Wine* as examples of 'growing old disgracefully', of how to enjoy life in old age. Physical and cognitive decline is not inevitable and old age must never be seen as a burden either to the person who is elderly or their families.

Often, post-retirement years are filled with activities that one did not have time for prior to retiring. As a nurse, you could explore ways that those with a learning disability could enjoy their old age and maintain their social links to their communities, such as:

- Frequent visits to cafés and pubs
- Engagement in sports or arts and craft type activities
- Engaging in voluntary work
- Engaging with the social and spiritual aspects of their chosen faith communities.

Many local swimming pools have sessions that cater for the needs of older people, for example, and it may be worth exploring how those with a learning disability could become involved in this activity.

Whilst there are a great many suitable and appropriate services for those who are elderly, there may well be a lack of similarly appropriate services for those who have a learning disability and who are elderly. This is particularly likely to be the case when working with those who have a profound and multiple learning disability (PMLD), although it is unlikely that those with a PMLD will live beyond their mid-60s due to the complexity and severity of their disabilities. Therefore, it may be useful to work with the local community learning disability team to design and create appropriate services that meet the holistic care and support needs of people like Jim or those with a PMLD, rather than trying to 'shoehorn' them into inappropriate existing services that are too generic to meet their needs.

10.7 **Conclusion**

This chapter has sought to highlight some of the health and care support needs of those who, like Jim, have a learning disability and age-related health conditions such as dementia. Some of these needs are likely to be very similar to those of any other elderly person, whilst others may be unique to those with a learning disability, particularly those with PMLD. The emphasis of nursing care and support must be to enable those who are elderly to enjoy their remaining years. Rather than having *'one foot in the grave'*, those with a learning disability and who are elderly should be able to enjoy being the *'last of the summer wine'*.

CHAPTER SUMMARY

Key points to take away from *Chapter 10*:
- ☑ Life expectancy of those with a learning disability is changing significantly, with increasing numbers reaching and living well into old age, both in terms of length of years and the quality of those years.
- ☑ Old age does not necessarily have to involve decreasing physical and mental health, with increasing numbers of very active people who are in their 70s and 80s.
- ☑ Those with a learning disability who do live into old age are likely to experience similar social and health issues as other elderly people, including sensory impairment, mobility problems, heart conditions, depression, arthritis and social isolation.
- ☑ Dementia is likely to be a major health and social issue, as around a third of all those with a learning disability are expected to develop dementia.
- ☑ The role of the nurse, nursing student and HCA is likely to be very challenging, as the possibility that those who have a learning disability reaching old age has only recently been planned and provided for.

Questions

Question 10.1   What is your understanding of 'normal' old age and associated health and social issues?

Question 10.2   Are there any differences in how those with a learning disability are likely to experience old age compared with their non-learning disabled peers?

Question 10.3   How would you explain the onset of old age and the physical and mental changes associated with old age to a person with a learning disability?

Question 10.4   As assessments are the basis of most if not all nursing care, how would you become aware of and assess the onset of the various health and sensory issues highlighted in this chapter?

Question 10.5   Is there a specialist dementia care / Admiral nurse for those with a learning disability? If so, how would you contact them for advice and assistance in supporting an elderly person with a learning disability?

Question 10.6   How would you promote living well and positively into old age whilst working with a person with a learning disability?

REFERENCES

Alzheimer's Society (undated) *Learning disability and the risk of developing dementia*. Available at: www.alzheimers.org.uk/about-dementia/types-dementia/learning-disability-risk-developing-dementia (accessed 4 January 2022).

Aylward, E., Burt, D., Thorpe, L., Lai, F. and Dalton, A. (1997) Diagnosis of dementia in individuals with intellectual disability. *Journal of Intellectual Disability Research*, **41**: 152–64.

Dementia UK (2019) *Learning disability and dementia*. Available at: www.dementiauk.org/get-support/maintaining-health-in-dementia/learning-disability-and-dementia/ (accessed 4 January 2022).

Diabetes UK (2018) *Why is improving diabetes care for people with a learning disability important?* Available at: www.diabetes.org.uk/resources-s3/2018-02/Improving%20care%20for%20peeople%20with%20diabetes%20and%20a%20learning%20disability%20-%20Fact%20sheet%201.pdf (accessed 4 January 2022).

Down's Syndrome Association (2018a) *Getting older*. Available at: www.downs-syndrome.org.uk/wp-content/uploads/2020/06/Ageing-Final-Format-5th-April-DSMIG.pdf (accessed 4 January 2022).

Down's Syndrome Association (2018b) *Dementia: Alzheimer's disease*. Available at: www.downs-syndrome.org.uk/wp-content/uploads/2020/06/2018.09.Alzheimers-Disease_DSMIG.pdf (accessed 4 January 2022).

Emerson, E. and Baines, S. (2010) *Health inequalities and people with learning disabilities in the UK: 2010*. Learning Disabilities Observatory.

Kiani, R. and Miller, H. (2010) Sensory impairment and intellectual disability. *Advances in Psychiatric Treatment*, **16(3)**: 228–35. Available at: www.cambridge.org/core/journals/advances-in-psychiatric-treatment/article/sensory-impairment-and-intellectual-disability/BDD74DB4E7DAD1ED57EC2D461DFFD06D (accessed 4 January 2022).

Neurotrauma Law Nexus (undated). *Neuroglossary*. Available at: www.neurolaw.com/neuroglossary/#d (accessed 4 January 2022).

NHS Digital (2020) *Health and care of people with learning disabilities: experimental statistics: 2018 to 2019*. Available at: https://digital.nhs.uk/data-and-information/publications/statistical/health-and-care-of-people-with-learning-disabilities/experimental-statistics-2018-to-2019 (accessed 4 January 2022).

NICE (2018) *Care and support of people growing older with learning disabilities* [NG96]. Available at: www.nice.org.uk/guidance/ng96 (accessed 4 January 2022).

Ouldred, E. and Bryant, C. (2008) 'The older adult: intellectual impairment and the dementias'. In Clark, L. and Griffiths, P. (eds) *Learning Disability and Other Intellectual Impairments*. John Wiley & Sons.

Prasher, V. (1995) Age-specific prevalence, thyroid dysfunction and depressive symptomology in adults with Down syndrome and dementia. *International Journal of Geriatric Psychiatry*, **10**: 25–31.

Royal College of Psychiatrists (2001) *DC–LD: diagnostic criteria for psychiatric disorders for use with adults with learning disabilities / mental retardation.* Gaskell (RCP).

Wallace, R. and Dalton, A. (2006) Clinicians' guide to physical health problems of older adults with Down syndrome. *Journal on Developmental Disabilities,* **12**:1 Down syndrome (supplement 1).

RESOURCES

Age UK: www.ageuk.org.uk (accessed 4 January 2022).

Dementia UK: www.dementiauk.org (accessed 4 January 2022).

Naidex: www.naidex.co.uk (accessed 4 January 2022).

NRS Healthcare: https://www.nrshealthcare.co.uk (accessed 4 January 2022).

Chapter 11
Dying, death and bereavement and people with a learning disability

AIMS AND LEARNING OUTCOMES

The aims of this chapter are to highlight aspects of:

- Dying
- Death, and
- Bereavement

as they apply to those with a learning disability.

By the end of this chapter, you will be able to discuss the various meanings of, and processes and rituals around:

- Dying
- Death, including the possible death of dreams, hopes and aspirations as a result of having a child with a learning disability
- Bereavement
- The roles of the nurse whilst supporting those with a learning disability and their families
- How to integrate some of the ideas within this chapter within your work.

SCENARIO 11.1: PAUL

Paul is a 55-year-old gentleman with a moderate learning disability who lives on his own but with support from a multi-agency team. His mother had died some ten years earlier and his 85-year-old father, with whom he is in regular and close contact, has been diagnosed with end-stage renal cancer and has been given only weeks to live.

Paul has an older sister, Stephanie, with whom he is also in close and frequent contact.

11.1 **Introduction**

As with many issues such as religion and human sexuality, dying, death and bereavement are hardly talked about in public and when they are, they are often couched in terms of misguided fear or misguided humour. However, it has been said that there are only three certainties in life: birth, taxation and death! Following on naturally from *Chapter 10*, which focused on elderly care and people with a learning disability, this chapter will focus on dying, death and bereavement.

Dying, death and bereavement are personal issues and experiences that, at some point in our lives, we will all have to acknowledge and face, possibly as nurses and certainly as ordinary people. Indeed, it is very likely that we will all have to face up to and acknowledge the death of our parents and grandparents. For some, it is the death of a sibling or a child that they have to face. Some people have to face the issues of dying, death and bereavement a lot sooner than others, whilst others do not encounter dying and death until they are themselves middle-aged or even elderly. Again, some people will experience dying and death at home surrounded by friends, family and the wider community, whilst others experience dying and death alone and in an alien environment such as a hospital ward. Those with a learning disability are no different. They, too, will have to face and accept dying, death and bereavement and sometimes face these alone.

11.2 **Dying**

Dying is a complex phenomenon as it encompasses a number of different issues:
- Dying as the end of life that is usually associated with old age
- Dying as a gradual process that could last from minutes to hours, days, weeks, months and even years
- Dying as a personal and even solitary experience
- Dying as a community experience
- Dying as journey to death
- The conflict between this journey and its inevitable conclusion and the fact that the person undertaking this journey is still very much alive.

PAUSE FOR THOUGHT 11.1

What does the process of dying mean for both you as a nurse and you as a person? Are there any differences? How would you explore these differences? Do these differences need to be reconciled and if so, how and why? Write down your observations and thoughts.

Dying is also likely to involve a number of different people and sets of relationships that could include:
- Parents watching and being involved in the dying process of their child who has a learning disability
- Parents who are, themselves, dying and are concerned as to how their disabled child would be able to cope with seeing their parent dying and what would happen to that child once the parent is dead

- Siblings and partners who are dying
- The person with a learning disability who is dying and who is concerned for their parent, sibling, partner or child
- The person with a learning disability who is aware that their parent, partner or sibling is dying. Those with a learning disability, according to Wiseman, Lowton and Noonan (2008) and the Nuffield Trust (2021), are more likely to be still living with their ageing parents and are thus more likely to witness, experience and be part of this dying process.

All of these relationships, dynamics and situations are different and will require different approaches in engaging, communicating and working with those who are involved in this dying process.

End of life care, be it for the parent as in *Scenario 11.1*, the sibling, the partner or the person who has a learning disability, is likely to be a major concern and is likely to involve a number of separate issues.

Where is end of life care to be delivered? Is end of life care to be delivered at hospital, in a care / nursing home, in a hospice or at the patient's own home (hospice at home)? These are very real issues which can have a major impact on Paul, his sister and their father. Indeed, is it appropriate to offer end of life care? End of life care is usually associated with cancer care or dementia; what if the patient does not have cancer or dementia? What if the patient is just dying of old age? Is a service that is geared up to meet the needs of those with various cancers needed or appropriate here?

Issues around appropriate pain relief and management are likely to surface and become increasingly important at this time (Wiseman, Lowton and Noonan, 2008; PCPLD Network, 2017). Those with a learning disability who are dying / receiving end of life care must be offered the same opportunity as everyone else to manage their pain levels through the use of medication or complementary therapies. Just because a person has a learning disability does not mean that they do not feel pain in the same way as anyone else. However, medication, its effects and side-effects must be closely monitored in order to prevent under- or overdosing errors.

Likewise, just because someone is dying does not mean that they are not still living. Therefore, opportunities for engaging in valued social and family activities should be offered but not forced upon the person.

Opportunities for the psychological and emotional preparation for the impending death of either the self or the family member must be offered with great sensitivity. Along with this must go the possibility of a need for personal reconciliation, either with the self or with others.

Many of those with a learning disability may hold and practise particular religious, cultural or spiritual beliefs. It may be appropriate to seek the support of the person's faith community and its leaders. This is particularly important when one realises that dying and death could be seen as forms of 'rites of passage' with their own religious, spiritual, cultural and community rites and rituals. Such religious and spiritual beliefs and practices may well provide emotional and psychological comfort, peace and acceptance within the person, preparing them for the 'ultimate journey' and thus must never be ignored or ridiculed. Consequently, those with a learning disability should be encouraged, if they so wish, to participate in religious services, rituals and liturgies, preferably at their usual place of worship and offer appropriate support if needed. By so doing, they participate in the ordinary life of their chosen faith community, and their faith community has the opportunity to participate in and celebrate the life of one of its members. (See *Chapter 14* for more on spirituality and religion).

ACTIVITY 11.1

List the various people mentioned in *Scenario 11.1*.

Beside each person, list their likely support needs and how you would set about meeting those needs.

11.3 Death

As with dying, death can be far from simple and can include a range of complex issues.

First, what is meant by death and when does death actually occur? According to Taylor (2019) death "is the cessation of all physical and chemical processes that occurs in all living organisms". Clinical death is the absence of a heartbeat, determined by a lack of a pulse and the cessation of breathing. Brain death is when there is no detectable brainstem activity as manifested by absolute unresponsiveness to all stimuli, absence of all spontaneous muscle activity, and two isoelectric electroencephalograms (the second test being 30 minutes after the first), all in the absence of hypothermia or intoxication by central nervous system depressants. The test for brain death is carried out by two different doctors and the time of death is that time when the second test has been carried out and the patient meets the criteria for brain death (Gardiner *et al.*, 2012).

One of the problems with this basic definition of death is the status of a person, who although to all intents and purposes would meet the criteria for being dead, is nonetheless 'kept alive' through artificial means such as being on a respirator. Is this person dead or alive? This is no mere philosophical or rhetorical question, as it underpins the ongoing debate around the therapeutic management of those in persistent vegetative states.

There are likely to be a variety of social, religious, spiritual or cultural rituals surrounding the death of a person. If death occurs in a hospital, it may be useful to contact the relevant hospital chaplain for advice and guidance for some of these rituals. For example, a person with a learning disability who is dying and is a Catholic might wish to receive the last rites of the church (what used to be called '*extreme unction*') before death occurs. If the person is able, they may wish to receive Holy Communion / Eucharist (*viaticum*) from a priest. Other religions and faith communities may have specific 'rites of passage' immediately prior to and after death.

If the death occurs in a hospital or care / nursing home, be it the death of a person who had a learning disability or their parent or family member, the last offices need to be carried out in accordance with local policies and practice. These are the 'last duties' carried out on the body of the deceased by the nurse:

- To prepare the deceased for the mortuary whilst respecting their cultural beliefs
- To comply with legislation, in particular where the death of a patient requires the involvement of a Coroner
- To minimise any risk of cross-infection to any relative, healthcare worker or other persons who may need to handle the deceased.

In *Scenario 11.1*, following the death of Paul's father, a number of duties would need to be carried out. These are likely to include:

- notifying other family members of the death
- arranging the funeral (contacting the undertakers and the dead person's faith community if appropriate)
- the reading and execution of any last will and testament
- notifying the Department for Work and Pensions and other relevant welfare benefits agencies so that any welfare benefits and/or pensions that the person received before their death are stopped
- notifying any banks or building societies regarding any bank accounts that the deceased may have held
- notifying any credit / debit card issuer regarding the cancellation of any cards that the deceased may have held
- notifying gas, water, electricity, broadband and phone providers of the death so that these services can be stopped.

Although Paul lives semi-independently, other people with a learning disability may live with their parents. If it is the parent who has died, the accommodation / residential needs of the person with a learning disability who may have been living with them must be met as a matter of urgency.

Given Paul's learning disability, it is likely that his sister, Stephanie, will have the responsibility for working through these generic duties. Therefore, any nurse or nursing student working with Paul would not be directly involved in carrying out these duties. Indeed, it may well be inappropriate for a nurse to do so. However, the multidisciplinary team, including nurses, may need to assist Paul to be involved in some of these duties, even if such involvement was limited to being informed of these duties, consulted about how they are to be carried out and knowing that his sister will be directly involved in this process. Paul will also need to be kept informed regarding the progress of these duties in a manner that best meets his emotional and communication needs at the time. Such involvement is likely to form a vital part of the bereavement process and Paul must not be excluded from this process simply because he has a learning disability.

During the days and weeks immediately after the death of a partner, a parent, a sibling or a child, most people are likely to 'operate on autopilot'; most people will therefore need time and assistance to work through the above duties, whether or not they have a learning disability.

11.4 Do not attempt cardiopulmonary resuscitation (DNACPR)

The issue of 'do not attempt cardiopulmonary resuscitation' (DNACPR) and those with a learning disability has risen very much to the fore since 2020, not only owing to the sensitive consent issues (whether those with a learning disability have the ability to give or withhold consent to DNACPR instructions). Learning Disability England (2018) published guidance on DNACPR and those with a learning disability, guidance which either was not read, not understood, not followed or sometimes ignored by medical doctors during the first Covid wave in 2020.

While the NHS is clear that people should not have a DNACPR on their record just because they have a learning disability, autism or both, there are often incidences in the national news about people with a learning disability or autism which comment on choices around death (Lintern, 2021). In December 2020, the CQC warned that inappropriate DNACPRs may have led to avoidable deaths and that many incorrect orders were likely to still be in place. In a letter dated March 2021, NHS England's National Medical Director Steve Powis, Chief Nursing Officer Ruth May and other health leaders stressed that doctors must consider the individual patient (Lintern, 2021; NHS England, 2021). The terms 'learning disability' and 'Down's syndrome' should never be a reason for issuing a DNACPR order (Learning Disability England, 2020) or be used to describe the underlying or only cause of death. Additionally, there was a huge scandal about the inappropriate issuing of DNACPRs to people with learning disabilities in hospitals as a 'blanket' practice (Tapper, 2021) and this gained a lot of traction in the media and resulted in some changes in general practice (Bloomer, 2021). These changes included new ethical guidance from the BMA to doctors indicating that the presence of a learning disability would "almost certainly not be a clinically relevant factor" in deciding a person's eligibility for treatment (BMA, 2020).

Whether the changes are enough to safeguard the basic human rights of those with a learning disability, namely the right to life and the right to fair and equal treatment, only time will tell. However, it is the role and duty of the nurse to be aware of and understand the issues involved and be an effective advocate for those in their care.

11.5 Bereavement

Given that this chapter has tended to focus on end of life issues, with dying and death as their inevitable conclusion, either of the person with a learning disability or their parent or sibling, bereavement may not be as simple as it may at first appear.

Imagine that you are a new parent who has just received the news that your child (be it born or yet to be born) has Down's syndrome. It is not unusual, even today, for such parents to mourn, to grieve for the child that they will not have and, along with that child, all the hopes, dreams and aspirations that parents would normally hold for a child. This is a very real form of bereavement and those so bereaved may need extra practical, emotional and psychological support to come to terms with the diagnosis. So, what is bereavement?

Bereavement is a process or journey by which one person mourns or grieves for the loss, usually through death, of another person and which can begin sometimes before the actual death (anticipatory grief) (Daly, 2017; Taee, 2020) and which can last for many years. This other person can be a family member, a friend or sometimes a well-known figure or personality where both the individual and the wider community collectively mourn or grieve for their death. An example of this is the national mourning for Diana, Princess of Wales, or Sir Winston Churchill at and after their respective funerals.

Stages of bereavement or grief are likely to include:
- shock or disbelief, mood swings, loss of concentration, sadness
- denial of the death or its effects on the person grieving
- anger at the loss of the person, either through death or through the diagnosis of disability; this anger can be directed either inwardly towards the self or outwardly towards either other people such as healthcare professionals or the deceased, or at God (however one perceives Him or Her)
- bargaining
- depression
- growing awareness, leading finally to
- acceptance and hope.

Parkes and Prigerson (2010) suggested two further additions: searching, either where the bereaved may have a sense of the dead person still being with them or a searching for meaning; and gaining a new identity (taking on roles previously carried out by the dead person in practical matters, personal mannerisms, characteristics and interests).

Grieving may not follow a straight path nor begin at the death of the person. Anticipatory grieving and bereavement may begin prior to death and may allow time for adjustment to that death to be made (Costello, 1999; Daly, 2017; Taee, 2020). Some people miss out on some of these stages, whilst others are likely to repeat stages already journeyed through. This journey broadly follows the model of bereavement formulated by Kübler-Ross (1969).

Someone with a learning disability such as Paul may well grieve in the same way as anyone else when they lose someone they love, whilst others will grieve in different ways. Sadly, they may also face more loss than other people, especially if they have friends with a learning disability whose life expectancy may be lower than average. Signs of grief can be difficult to spot and will be different for each person; some people may get angry, while others may become withdrawn or even destructive. Grief and bereavement can be complicated by:
- the nature of the relationship that the bereaved had with the deceased
- whether the death was sudden, unexpected or untimely

- circumstances where many bereavements may have happened together or in quick succession, such as may occur in a serious road traffic or rail accident
- how the deaths occurred
- when a death re-evokes an insufficiently mourned previous death, as may be the case with Paul now that both his parents are dead
- where there is no family or social support network.

As Paul journeys through bereavement his behaviour may change as a result of being unable to express his feelings verbally. Such changes may include (CWP, 2017):

- clinging
- reluctance to leave the house
- uncharacteristic incontinence
- self-injury
- restlessness
- aches and pains (often muscular or abdominal)
- changes in sleep pattern alongside not wanting to sleep on his own
- changes in or loss of appetite
- apathy or tiredness
- minor illness
- clumsiness and accidents.

CWP (2017) suggests that those with a learning disability have often been given fewer opportunities to find out about death and bereavement and so may take longer to journey through and resolve their grief over the death of a family member or friend.

11.6 The role of the nurse

Jill works part time in a GP practice and part time in a community health centre as a healthcare assistant within a community health team. Jill has been asked to work with and support not only Paul but also his sister Stephanie during the period before and after their father's death.

The roles of the nurse when supporting those with a learning disability who are journeying through dying, death and bereavement can be very challenging yet fulfilling.

- Jill would be well advised to contact the community learning disability team for advice and assistance in providing appropriate support to Paul and his sister during the periods before and after the death of their father.
- Jill will need to understand that Paul's emotional and psychological needs and the ways that he may experience and express anticipatory grief are likely to be different to those of his sister Stephanie (CWP, 2017). Such differences are likely to impact upon how needs are met. A 'one size fits all' approach would be inappropriate, not good practice and may cause further problems and even harm to both Paul and Stephanie.
- Paul and Stephanie must be allowed and helped to prepare for the death of their father in their own ways. This must include giving Paul the opportunity to say

'goodbye' to his father if he wishes to (CWP, 2017). This is his right and this right must never be taken away from him.

- Paul may express confusion, fear and even anticipatory grief through changes in his behaviour, and Jill must anticipate these behavioural changes and seek assistance in dealing appropriately with them. Historically, those with a learning disability were often not informed of the death of their parent or sibling until some time after the death had occurred, and occasionally not even then (CWP, 2017). The person with a learning disability did not have the chance to say 'goodbye', to be involved in social and religious rituals around dying and death, to attend the funeral or to visit the cemetery. This has often impacted negatively upon the person's behaviour, behaviour that was then wrongly managed.

- Jill will need to explain to Paul in simple and honest language what is happening to his father, in terms of the dying and death processes; she must not use euphemisms around dying and death, such as referring to death as 'falling asleep', as a 'loss' or saying that the deceased is now in heaven (CWP, 2017). This may suggest that those who are dead can be re-awakened or that those who are asleep may be dead. Paul may thus be afraid to sleep at night. 'Death as loss' may suggest that whatever has been lost can be found. Paul may come to believe that the cemetery where his father is buried is in, or is itself, heaven.

- Jill should explain that death happens to everyone and it is when the body has stopped working and cannot be mended. Jill also needs to explain to Paul that his dead father can no longer feel any pain. There are resources that are available around dying, death and bereavement that may be useful (see Resources section at the end of this chapter).

- Paul should be allowed to view the body of his father if he wishes, but must not be forced to do so.

- Paul must be allowed to participate alongside his sister in arranging his father's funeral if he wishes. Jill should explain what happens at a funeral and burial or cremation and the roles that Paul may like to take. It may be useful to seek advice from the undertakers and/or the dead person's faith community as to specific roles that Paul could take during the funeral service.

- Paul must be encouraged to talk about his father and listened to with care and compassion. Paul may wish to talk to someone from outside his family and immediate circle of friends and may need support to enable this (CWP, 2017). A drama, music or art group may be useful in enabling Paul to come to terms with the death of his father and express his grief.

- Likewise, designing with Paul a small and simple memorial garden, garden of memories or planting of a memorial tree, both as an activity and as a simple ceremony involving Paul's sister and friends, could be encouraged. Paul should be assisted to maintain his relationship and contact with his sister Stephanie and other members of his family.

- As this aspect of nursing work is likely to be emotionally and mentally draining, Jill must be offered appropriate professional support through supervision, ongoing training and development and, if needed, counselling.

11.7 Conclusion

The death of a loved family member or friend can often be a very painful and sad experience for anyone; particularly so if they have a learning disability. Yet it can also be a time of great challenge, peace, self-discovery and growth for the individual and those around them. Either way, dying, death and bereavement are not journeys that a person should embark upon alone. After all, this is a journey that all of us, regardless of who we are, will have to take at some point in our lives.

CHAPTER SUMMARY

Key points to take away from *Chapter 11*:

- ✅ Dying, death and bereavement are normal life experiences that we all have to engage with, either as nurses and/or as people.
- ✅ Dying is a journey to death whilst the person is still very much alive.
- ✅ Death is "the cessation of all physical and chemical processes that occurs in all living organisms".
- ✅ Bereavement is a process or journey by which one person mourns or grieves for the loss, usually through death, of another person and which can begin sometimes before the actual death (anticipatory grief).
- ✅ The person with a learning disability will and must be allowed to experience dying, death and bereavement in their own way and in their own time and is likely to need practical, emotional and psychological support in order to engage with these journeys appropriately.

Questions

Question 11.1	What is your understanding of end of life care? How would you support a person with a learning disability whose parent or sibling was reaching the end of their life?
Question 11.2	Given the brief definition of death above, is this too simplistic a definition and, if so, how would you define death? What aspects of death are missing from the above definition?
Question 11.3	How would you support a person with a learning disability in the event of the death of a parent, sibling, partner or friend?
Question 11.4	What do you consider to be the ongoing needs of a person with a learning disability in the months and years after the death of a parent, sibling or friend? How would you go about meeting those needs?

REFERENCES

Bloomer, A. (2021) *Do not resuscitate orders and learning disability: where are we now?* Learning Disability Today. Available at: www.learningdisabilitytoday.co.uk/do-not-resuscitate-orders-and-learning-disability-where-are-we-now (accessed 4 January 2022).

British Medical Association (2020) *COVID-19: ethical issues when demand for life-saving treatment is at capacity.* Available at: www.bma.org.uk/advice-and-support/covid-19/ethics/covid-19-ethical-issues-when-demand-for-life-saving-treatment-is-at-capacity (accessed 4 January 2022).

Cheshire and Wirral Partnership (CWP) NHS Trust (2017) *Bereavement and Learning Disabilities: a guide for carers.* Available at: www.cwp.nhs.uk/media/3508/bereavement-and-learning-disabilities-a-guide-for-carers-master.pdf (accessed 4 January 2022).

Costello, J. (1999) Anticipatory grief: coping with the impending death of a partner. *International Journal of Palliative Nursing,* **5(5)**: 223–31.

Daly, E. (2017) *Anticipatory grief: when someone you love is seriously ill.* Counselling Directory. Available at: www.counselling-directory.org.uk/memberarticles/anticipatory-grief-when-someone-you-love-is-seriously-ill (accessed 4 January 2022).

Gardiner, B., Shemie, S., Manara, A. and Opdam, H. (2012) International perspective on the diagnosis of death. *BJA: British Journal of Anaesthesia*, **108**: i14–i28.

Kübler-Ross, E. (1969) *On Death and Dying.* Routledge.

Learning Disability England (2018) *DNACPR Support Pack.* Available at: www.learningdisabilityengland.org.uk/wp-content/uploads/2020/06/DNACPR-Support-Pack.pdf (accessed 4 January 2022).

Learning Disability England (2020) *DNR: A guide for understanding your rights and challenging decisions.* Available at: www.learningdisabilityengland.org.uk/news/latest-news/dnar-a-guide-for-understanding-your-rights-and-challenging-decisions/ (accessed 4 January 2022).

Lintern, S. (2021) *Doctors warned again over unlawful use of do not resuscitate orders.* Available at: www.independent.co.uk/news/health/covid-do-not-resuscitate-nhs-b1816413.html (accessed 4 January 2022).

NHS England (2021) Available at: www.england.nhs.uk/coronavirus/wp-content/uploads/sites/52/2020/04/C1146-dnacpr-and-people-with-a-learning-disability-and-or-autism.pdf (accessed 4 January 2022).

Nuffield Trust (2021) *Adults with learning disabilities who live in their own home or with their family.* Available at: www.nuffieldtrust.org.uk/resource/adults-with-learning-disabilities-who-live-in-their-own-home-or-with-their-family (accessed 4 January 2022).

Palliative Care for People with Learning Disabilities Network (2017) *Delivering high quality end of life care for people who have a learning disability.* Available at: www.england.nhs.uk/wp-content/uploads/2017/08/delivering-end-of-life-care-for-people-with-learning-disability.pdf (accessed 4 January 2022).

Parkes, C. and Prigerson, H. (2010) *Bereavement: studies of grief in adult life*, 4th edition. Penguin.

Taee, K. (2020) *What is anticipatory grief?* Available at: www.mariecurie.org.uk/talkabout/articles/what-is-anticipatory-grief/271278 (accessed 4 January 2022).

Tapper, J. (2021) *Fury at 'do not resuscitate' notices given to Covid patients with learning disabilities.* Available at: www.theguardian.com/world/2021/feb/13/new-do-not-resuscitate-orders-imposed-on-covid-19-patients-with-learning-difficulties (accessed 4 January 2022).

Taylor, J. (ed.) (2019) *Baillière's Dictionary for Nurses and Healthcare Workers*, 27th edition. Elsevier.

Wiseman, T., Lowton, K. and Noonan, I. (2008) 'Transitions in the ageing population'. In Clarke, L. and Griffiths, P. (2008) *Learning Disability and Other Intellectual Impairments*. John Wiley & Sons.

RESOURCES

Books Beyond Words: https://booksbeyondwords.co.uk/ (accessed 4 January 2022).
The following books may be useful:
- *When Dad Died*
- *When Mum Died*
- *When Somebody Dies*
- *Am I Going to Die?*

Hospice UK: www.hospiceuk.org/our-campaigns/dying-matters (accessed 4 January 2022).

Marie Curie: www.funeralguide.co.uk/help-resources/bereavement-support/helping-the-bereaved/supporting-someone-with-a-learning-disability-through-grief (accessed 4 January 2022).

Mencap: www.mencap.org.uk/advice-and-support/dealing-bereavement (accessed 4 January 2022).

National Institute for Health and Care Excellence (NICE) has a range of useful resources. Go to the Evidence search page and type 'death and dying learning disabilities' in the search bar: www.evidence.nhs.uk (accessed 4 January 2022).

Chapter 12
Care and support for those who are informal caregivers

AIMS AND LEARNING OUTCOMES

The aims of this chapter are to highlight:

- The meaning of informal caregiving

- The demographics of informal caregiving

- The experiences of those who are informal caregivers

- Caregiver legislation

- The roles of the nurse in supporting informal caregivers.

By the end of this chapter you will be able to understand and discuss:

- The meaning of informal caregiving

- The personal experiences of those caring for a family member who has a learning disability

- The existence and impact of caregiver legislation on the lives of caregivers

- The role of the nurse in supporting those who are informal caregivers, integrating some of these roles in your work.

PAUSE FOR THOUGHT 12.1

"I shouldn't have to spend my life proving that my son can't do things, to get the support my family needs to help him do things for himself."

12.1 Introduction

Up to now, the focus of this book has been on those with a learning disability and their needs. In previous generations, those with a learning disability lived within specialist learning disability hospitals such as South Ockendon hospital in Essex, where I trained as a nurse in the last third of the 1980s. When these hospitals finally closed their doors in the 1990s, those with a learning disability were cared for within small community-based homes, a practice that was in line with official government policy of the day.

As a result of the closure of these long-stay hospitals, many people with a learning disability now live either on their own with support or with their own families, the latter being a reality that may place an extra share of caring responsibility on these families. Therefore, the focus of this chapter will shift to these families, these 'informal caregivers', and their experiences of caring for a person with a learning disability. Whilst much of this chapter will focus on issues that are pertinent to all caregivers rather than caregivers of those with a learning disability, parallels and implications will be made apparent for those caring for a family member who has a learning disability. I am indebted here to the *British Journal of Healthcare Assistants* for its kind permission in allowing the use of definitions and statistics as they had been used in a series of articles written by me on caregivers.

12.2 What is 'informal caregiving'?

There are a number of issues around not so much the definition of informal care and carers but rather the language that is used. Some carers get rather annoyed at being called 'informal', saying that there is nothing informal about what they do. Often, the term 'caregiver' is preferred to that of 'informal carer' and will be used throughout this chapter. So, what is this thing called 'care' and who are 'caregivers' anyway? What is the difference between these and 'formal care' and 'formal carers'?

Formal carers	Caregivers/informal carers
People who are employed, paid, trained and often regulated to provide care to another person. This will include care professionals such as doctors, nurses, HCAs, social workers, professionals allied to medicine and religious ministers. Formal care is any care services that are provided by these care professionals in their professional lives.	People who provide care and support to a family member such as a grandparent, a parent, a partner, a sibling or a child with a disability or a friend in any care setting. This care is provided free, without pay, regulation and often without training, although there are an increasing number and variety of workshops, conferences and short training courses relevant and available for caregivers. Examples of caregivers include parents, partners, children, siblings, aunts, uncles, grandparents and friends.

A more formal definition of caregivers may look like the following:

"A carer is anyone who cares, unpaid, for a friend or family member who due to illness, disability, a mental health problem or an addiction cannot cope without their support. Anyone could be a carer: a 15-year-old girl looking after a parent with an alcohol problem, a 40-year-old man caring for his partner who has terminal cancer, or an 80-year-old woman looking after her husband who has Alzheimer's disease." (Carers Trust, undated)

In many ways, the roles of the caregiver and the care professional overlap and it will not be unusual for caregivers to carry out nursing roles such as wound or pain management. It is not unusual for caregivers to be formal care professionals as well.

Based on statistics obtained from the 2011 population census, there were around 6.5 million caregivers in the UK, which was 11% of the UK population, given a population of 60 million between the four countries of the UK (England, Scotland, Wales and Northern Ireland) (Carers UK, 2014). The latest population survey was carried out in 2021, except in Scotland where it was postponed because of the Covid pandemic. It can fairly safely be assumed that the number of those who are caregivers would have increased in line with the UK population. The current UK population is about 65 million, of which around 11% are caregivers, which gives a caregiver population of about 7 million. Caregivers come from both genders, with a gender split of around 58% female and 42% male (Carers UK, 2019b). Caregivers come from all ethnic backgrounds and cultures and from all ages from young children aged 7 or 8 who are caring for a sick or disabled sibling or parent to people who are in their 80s or 90s caring for a partner with dementia. Caregivers come from all social backgrounds: from the former Prime Minister David Cameron, who cared for his son before he died in 2009, to those living anonymously below the 'poverty line'. Those with a learning disability may also be caregivers looking after a disabled or elderly parent.

- Around 11% of the UK population are caregivers.
- Around 58% of caregivers are female and 42% are male.
- 64% of all caregivers are caring for more than 50 hours a week. This suggests that in just nine years the proportion of unpaid carers providing 50 hours of care or more per week has almost tripled since the 2011 Census (23%) (Carers Trust, 2020).
- 68% of all caregivers are of working age (Carers UK, 2019b).
- Primary school-aged children can become caregivers.
- 1.4 million (20%) of all caregivers give up paid employment in order to fulfil their caring responsibilities. Carer's Allowance was £67.60 a week in 2021 and to qualify for Carer's Allowance, the caregiver must be caring for at least 35 hours a week and can only earn an extra £128 per week (after tax and National Insurance has been deducted) through paid employment. It must also be kept in mind both that Carer's Allowance is taxable and not tax-free, and that the weekly amount will rise each year. This could, therefore, potentially have a significant impact upon family income and could even lead to family poverty, as this amounts to an annual income of around £10 000. To put this into perspective, this means that the caregiver 'earns' less than £2 per hour from the Carer's Allowance, bearing in mind that the national minimum wage in 2021 was £8.91 an hour for those aged 23 and over (HM Government, 2021). For those who care for 70 hours or more a week as some do, the hourly 'pay' rate (Carer's Allowance) is less than £1. There is an anecdotal suggestion that those in paid employment often find that their promotion prospects are hindered, although this would be illegal under the 2010 Equalities Act.
- In over half of households with working-age carers looking after their partners, no one in that household is in paid employment (Carers UK, 2019b). For people who care for just a few hours each week there is no evidence that care has an impact on labour market participation. Lower intensity carers actually have a

higher employment rate than people who provide no informal care: 77% of lower intensity carers (people caring for less than 10 hours per week) were in work over the three years to 2013/14, compared to an employment rate for non-carers of 74%. But as care levels increase employment decreases, with a clear impact on full-time employment. Among people providing 35 hours of care or more each week, 40% were in employment (Aldridge and Hughes, 2016). At least 1.2 million carers are now living in poverty across the UK, whilst half of working-age carers live in a household where no one is in paid employment. Compounding this situation, on average, 600 carers a day are having to leave work to provide unpaid care (Carers UK, undated).

- The amount that is saved to the UK economy by carers is £132 billion annually (Carers UK, 2019a). For every hour per day every day that is spent in caring, the caregiver saves the UK economy £6570 a year. Thus, if a caregiver cares for 50 hours a week (7 hours per day every day) the annual amount of money that is saved to the UK economy becomes £46 000.
- The amount that was saved to the UK economy by caregivers was £135 billion during the Covid-19 pandemic. This amounts to £370 million each and every day.
- 7% of caregivers care for someone with a learning disability (Ouldred and Bryant, 2008).
- An estimated 25% of those with a learning disability are not known to social services (Ouldred and Bryant, 2008).
- FPLD (undated) provides further basic details of informal carer and learning disability statistics.
- The 'State of Caring Survey' carried out by Carers UK (Carers UK, 2019a) suggests caregivers were twice as likely to experience anxiety as those who were not carers. Carers who have been caring for over 15 years were more likely to report poorer health, with 27% describing their mental health as bad or very bad. Carers looking after disabled children under the age of 18 reported significantly poorer mental health – 36% described their mental health as bad or very bad.
- Although these statistics relate to data based largely on the 2011 census, a policy briefing published by Carers UK (Carers UK, 2019b) provides updated projections and estimates and also makes the point that the carer population is not static.

ACTIVITY 12.1

You have been asked to present a short teaching session to your colleagues on caregivers. Present written data in the form of a table, infographic or 2–3 presentation slides around the numbers, percentages, gender and ages along with cost savings to the national economy of those giving informal care, which could be used in such a teaching session.

12.3 Experiences of those who are caregivers

People who care for a family member who has learning disabilities face many of the same challenges as those in other family carer roles, but with distinct differences. Many people with learning disabilities depend on family support all their lives, regardless of where they live, or until the carer dies (Gressmann, 2014).

During many informal conversations held by this author with caregivers over a number of years in a number of environments, views regarding how these caregivers perceived the input and care by care professionals were aired. All of these views were anecdotal in nature and were written down as and when they occurred naturally, although those making these anecdotal comments were aware that I was a nurse. Most of these care professionals were nurses. Whilst a small number of these comments were positive and complimentary of the care professionals whom caregivers had engaged with, most, however, were angry and frustrated. Many of these conversations can be distilled down to the comments that are contained in the following boxes. Whilst the vast majority of these comments appear negative, no attempt to edit these has been made, as these represent the raw and often painful but real experiences of caregivers. To edit these comments would downplay and invalidate these experiences. All these comments were made by people who are caregivers who are supporting and caring for their family members or friends whilst accessing healthcare services.

> "The support that I get from nurses, care staff, doctors, in fact all the ward staff is absolutely brilliant. They understand my son's needs, my needs as his father and have time for him and are able to communicate well with him and me."

Although the anecdotal comments that form the basis of this section were collected over a number of years from quite a large number of people, the above comment appears to be a rarity in its positive view of the support that a caregiver received from care professionals, particularly nurses.

> "When my son, who has autism, developed tonsillitis (which was a common occurrence) I phoned my GP for antibiotics. The agency GP practice nurse whom I spoke to said that it was flu, could not be bothered to look at my son's medical notes and put the phone down on me when I asked her to look at and read them."
>
> "My GP does not want to know."
>
> "Despite me being very stressed and my local GP practice nurse knowing that I am a full-time caregiver, this practice nurse either did not realise and understand how stressful and sometimes lonely being a caregiver is or just could not be bothered. Either way, she passed up an excellent opportunity to ask how I was coping and, indeed, *whether* I was coping."
>
> "The GP practice receptionist gave me inaccurate information regarding a query that I had regarding medication. Despite the stress that this caused me, the receptionist could not be bothered and came across as not caring or giving a damn about the harmful consequences of her actions."

These four comments highlight a perception, perhaps all too common, by some caregivers that they are isolated and ignored by their GPs or GP practice nurses. However, increasing numbers of GP practices are compiling a register of caregivers within their patch and promoting caregiver assessments and support for those on this register. Therefore, the support experienced by caregivers who access GP services should improve.

"I receive no respite care."

"I am on-call 24/7."

"There is nothing left of me."

"I have no support at all from anyone. I care 24/7 for my autistic adult daughter who left supported living because of abuse and neglect. I have had no help in four months. I live alone, am disabled myself and have been left to meet every single one of my daughter's needs, from accommodation, to mental health (she was suicidal when she first came here) and everything else. Her SW [social worker] promised at least outreach support but as yet none has materialised. I have finally managed to get her some talking therapy but it is a fight for everything and I have no one supporting me. There is almost no possibility of independent housing for her so no help with accommodation, no local groups or activities for her so all her leisure and social needs have to be met by me, she was very ill when she returned so her physical health has required a huge amount of work and I have had not one second's help with that from anyone. I'm at breaking point but there's nothing out there."

Again, these four comments that speak of tiredness and exhaustion are all too common in the lives of caregivers. Such exhaustion can and in many instances does lead to burnout and declining physical, emotional and mental health in the caregiver, and consequently to a decrease in ability to care. It can also lead to mistakes being carried out by the caregiver, mistakes that can have significant consequences for the cared for.

"The nurses do not understand."

"The nurses do not have the time to read my daughter's notes."

"I have to do everything for my daughter when she has to go into hospital."

Nursing and medical staff do not appear to have the training or ability to provide compassionate understanding, care and support to those with a learning disability and their caregivers within NHS facilities such as a hospital ward. Consider whether appropriate, correct and safe care and treatment can be offered to any patient, whether learning disabled or not, if that patient's care/case notes are not read.

"I received only 15 minutes' training on how to give morphine injections to my adult son who has cancer."

"I have attended a one-day workshop on autism and I know everything that there is to know about this disorder" (comment made by a social worker in the presence of a parent of a teenager with autism)

These comments relate to issues around appropriate training for both caregivers and care professionals. In relation to the first of these, consider how long it takes to train a student nurse to administer paracetamol to a patient without being supervised.

Inappropriate training of care professionals and caregivers could lead to very unsafe practices (15 minutes' training on how to administer morphine).

"When I accompanied my daughter who has a learning disability, and who was threatening to overdose on prescribed painkillers, to our local A&E department at no point did the A&E nursing staff take me to one side and allow me to talk, to unburden myself, to cry, let alone give me any support."

"There is very little out there to help me."

"There is no place to rest and have a tea or coffee whilst in hospital supporting my daughter."

These three comments speak of the caregivers' need for emotional and psychological support for themselves, care and support which should be freely available, and their near-desperation when such support is not available or offered. These comments speak also of missed opportunities by nursing staff to reach out to, support and assist caregivers.

"No one communicates."

"The nursing and medical staff do not ask me or listen to me. I am not included in the care of my son despite the fact that I know my son and his needs better than they do."

"I am ignored by the nursing staff whilst I am with my son in hospital."

The key points here appear to be the feeling of being ignored, of not being listened to by care professionals or included as a valued member of the multidisciplinary care team, and a lack of communication between care professionals and caregivers.

However, it may be that these remarks are more universal, standing as a sad comment on how many caregivers are viewed and treated by some care professionals, and indicate a widespread need for improvement across all services and support provided to those with a learning disability and their caregivers.

ACTIVITY 12.2

Take one issue from each of the above boxes, with the exception of the first box (you should have six issues). Write brief notes on how you would go about improving the caregiver's experience in each of these issues. Use this as a learning/teaching opportunity during staff team meetings while you are on placement. Ask colleagues to engage in this activity, choosing different issues and then compare notes. Remember: change what you can, understand and refer on to others what you cannot change and know and understand the difference between the two!

12.4 Caregiver legislation and strategy

There has been over the past three decades a growing realisation that the needs of caregivers go largely unrecognised and unmet. In order to address this, a number of

Acts of Parliament have been passed. All of these can be downloaded, free of charge, from the official Houses of Parliament website (see Resources) and www.legislation. gov.uk/.

Carers (Recognition and Services) Act 1995: The Carers Act 1995, as it is more commonly known, came into force on 1 April 1996 and was the first such legislation in the UK that specifically recognised the existence of caregivers. Under this Parliamentary Act, individuals who provide or intend to provide a substantial amount of care on a regular basis are entitled to request an assessment of their ability to carry out and to continue to carry out that care. This assessment is carried out at the same time and was likely to form a part of the service user assessment.

Carers and Disabled Children Act 2000: The Carers and Disabled Children Act 2000 applies to caregivers over 16 years of age and made the following principal changes to the existing 1995 Carers Act:

- It gave local councils mandatory duties to support caregivers by providing services to caregivers directly.
- It gave caregivers the right to an assessment independent of the person they care for.
- It empowered local authorities to make direct payments to caregivers.
- It enabled councils to support flexibility in provision of short breaks through the short breaks voucher scheme.

Carers (Equal Opportunities) Act 2004: The first key area of this Act was that it imposed a duty on local and health authorities not only to provide caregivers with an assessment (the 1995 Act) that was independent of any assessment, needs and wishes of the cared for (the 2000 Act), but also to inform caregivers of their rights to such an assessment. The problem still remained, however, that local social services, councils and health authorities were largely unaware of exactly who or where the caregivers were. That was due, in part, to caregivers not making themselves known as such to local social services or GP practices. The second key issue within the Act was the recognition that many, if not most, caregivers would like and even need paid employment and a social life outside of their caregiving role.

Carers at the Heart of 21st Century Families and Communities 2008: This strategy paper was expected to deliver genuine equality and recognition for caregivers:

- Caregivers to have a life of their own outside of caring
- Caregivers to be supported so they did not suffer financial hardship as a result of their caregiver responsibilities
- Caregivers to be respected as expert care providers
- A 'social contract' called for the setting out of the responsibilities and expectations of the State, employers and caregivers
- Caregivers to be supported to remain physically and mentally healthy.

Recognised, Valued and Supported: Next Steps for the Carers Strategy 2010: This strategy paper set out four years of actions to support the carers strategy.

- The government to work with caregivers and caregiver organisations to ease the burden of caregiving
- Provision of £40 million over the four years (which works out at £6.66 in total over the four years or £1.66 each year for each of the 6 million caregivers in the UK)
- Four priority areas were identified, in collaboration with caregivers and caregiver organisations:
  - supporting those with caring responsibilities to identify themselves as caregivers
  - enabling those with caregiver responsibilities to fulfil their employment and educational potential
  - personalised support for both cared for and caregiver
- Supporting caregivers to remain mentally and physically well.

Equality Act 2010: An Act to make provision to require Ministers of the Crown and others to have regard to the desirability of reducing socioeconomic inequalities; to reform and harmonise equality law and restate the greater part of the enactments relating to discrimination and harassment related to certain personal characteristics; to enable certain employers to be required to publish information about the differences in pay between male and female employees; to prohibit victimisation in certain circumstances; to require the exercise of certain functions to eliminate discrimination and other prohibited conduct; to increase equality of opportunity; to amend the law relating to rights and responsibilities in family relationships; and for connected purposes.

Chapter 1: Protected characteristics
1. Age
2. Disability
3. Marriage and civil partnerships
4. Race
5. Religion or belief
6. Sex, sexual orientation and gender reassignment

Chapter 2: Prohibited behaviour
1. Direct discrimination
2. Indirect discrimination

Care Act 2014: An Act to make provision to reform the law relating to care and support for adults and the law relating to support for carers; to make provision about safeguarding adults from abuse or neglect; to make provision about care standards; to establish and make provision about Health Education England; to establish and make provision about the Health Research Authority; to make provision about integrating care and support with health services; and for connected purposes.

The law requires local and health authorities to:
- promote individual wellbeing
- prevent needs for care and support
- promote integration of care and support with health services
- provide information and advice

- promote diversity and quality in provision of services
- cooperate generally and in specific cases
- provide assessments and relevant support services for caregivers
- provide assessments and relevant support for adults with care needs.

It could be argued from the above that legislative support for caregivers began from a somewhat grudging social service-led assessment of caregivers' needs and abilities as an aspect of the assessment of the patient or service user, with the duty to request such an assessment resting solely with the caregiver. However, the caregiver was unlikely to ask for an assessment of their own needs if they did not know that they could or how they could. Caregiver legislation as it now stands states that the caregiver has the right to have an assessment of their needs independent of any assessment of the person they care for and independent of the wishes of the cared for. Local authorities have a legal duty to inform caregivers of their rights and to inform them in such a way that meets the information requirements of the caregiver. However, this is not the same as those caregiver needs, once assessed, being appropriately met! The DHSC (2018) published a *Carers action plan* which covered the years 2018–2020 which promised a range of improvements to existing caregiver support service. However, it is debatable how much of this action plan has been implemented and whether informal caregivers have noticed any appreciable difference in the quality of their lives.

ACTIVITY 12.3

Obtain and read the relevant sections of the Equality Act (2010), the Care Act (2014) (see the Resources section for relevant websites) and related carer strategies. Are these still 'fit for purpose'? How could they be improved?

You may like to follow this activity up by considering the possibility of lobbying and seeking the support of your MP in order to raise caregiver improvement issues.

12.5 The roles of the nurse

SCENARIO 12.1

Jill, whom we met towards the end of *Chapter 9*, works at a GP practice as a healthcare assistant and at a local community health centre. Whilst working within these settings with a number of patients and service users who have a learning disability, she comes into regular contact with a number of their families. Consequently, Jill has developed an interest in supporting these families to meet their own needs.

The Foundation for People with Learning Disabilities (undated) suggested that 7 out of 10 families caring for someone with profound and multiple learning disabilities have reached or have come close to 'breaking point' because of a lack of short break services. Many caregivers have historically stated that there is a need for emotional support, respite breaks, access to support groups, independent advocacy and advice regarding planning for the future. Whilst these make for good starting points, where exactly does Jill start?

A good starting point for Jill would be to access Carers UK (www.carersuk.org) and the Carers Trust (www.carers.org) for a working knowledge of:

- caregiver definitions and the differences between 'informal caregivers' and care professionals
- caregiver statistics such as prevalence, gender mix, age range, likelihood of comorbid health issues, etc.
- the main issues that are likely to affect caregivers, such as their health, access to services, employment, sociopolitical issues, financial wellbeing, social isolation, care providers communicating and working with each other, ongoing 'professional' training, etc.
- access to caregiver surveys, the response to which rarely makes easy reading
- caregiver legislation and associated national, regional and local strategies.

Jill could become a member of either or both of these two organisations as a way of keeping herself informed and up to date with current issues affecting caregivers, and local caregiver support organisations are usually very willing to do short presentations to care professionals in order to raise awareness and understanding. Jill should not forget that those with a learning disability may also be caregivers themselves, as well as being care recipients, in so far as they could be the primary caregiver for an elderly or disabled parent. As such they are likely to need extra support both as a person with a learning disability and as a caregiver.

On a practical level, Jill could do the following:

- Ensure that all GP and health centre appointments and appointment times, whether for the caregiver or the person cared for, are based upon the needs of the caregiver and the cared for rather than the needs of the service. This will also include ensuring that enough time is given to the consultation so that the caregiver feels listened to and not rushed. A double appointment may be appropriate here. This would be in line with understanding and making 'reasonable adjustments' as required by the Equality Act 2010.
- Ask the right questions in the right way and at the right time of the caregiver and make time to listen carefully to the answers. If the right questions are not asked, do not be surprised if the right answers are not forthcoming. Remember that the caregiver is likely to know more about caring for someone with a learning disability than Jill does! Remember also that the caregiver is likely to have needs, many of which may be unmet. Make every contact count! This applies regardless of clinical or care setting.
- Provide clear, accurate and up-to-date information regarding a wide range of issues that are pertinent to caregivers and in a format that is accessible for caregivers. This format could be either written or verbal, in English or a wide variety of community languages, from academic journal articles to 'easy read'.
- Be involved in caregiver assessments as part of a multidisciplinary team.
- Advocate on behalf of family caregivers in the provision of equipment, carers' grants, welfare benefits and respite care, amongst many others.

- Help to set up and facilitate caregiver support groups at the health centre where she works. This may simply involve booking the meeting room and speakers, providing basic admin support and refreshments, and being available to answer caregivers' questions.
- Ensure that channels of communication include, where and when appropriate, the caregiver, keeping in mind the need and requirement for confidentiality to be maintained.

Those nurses who work in surgical or medical wards or, for that matter, any ward within a general acute hospital could offer caregivers who spend significant time at the hospital caring for and supporting their family member or friend the opportunity to use the staff room for comfort breaks. After all, you would not like the idea of working an entire shift without taking a coffee break; neither do caregivers! It might also be possible to lobby on behalf of carers for concessionary parking rates, staff discounts in the hospital catering outlets, and so on.

12.6 **Conclusion**

Caregivers can often be faced with a daunting task that could involve working or being available '24/7' and often without appropriate support from health and social care professionals. Yet, it can often be these same care professionals to whom caregivers turn for help and support and it can often be these care professionals who identify that caregivers are in need of support and what that support is likely to be. If in doubt, remember that the NMC's code of professional conduct places a professional duty on all nurses to communicate and work collaboratively with all members of the multidisciplinary team including patients/service users and their families.

CHAPTER SUMMARY

Key points to take away from *Chapter 12*:
- ☑ There are 7 million caregivers in the UK, i.e. 11% of the current UK population. A caregiver is a person of any age, adult or child, who provides unpaid support to a partner, child, relative or friend who could not manage to live independently or whose health or wellbeing would deteriorate without this help.
- ☑ Many caregivers are likely to have negative experiences of support and care at the hands of care professionals.
- ☑ There are a number of Parliamentary Acts that serve to meet the diverse needs of caregivers.
- ☑ The role of the nurse includes listening to and providing accurate information to caregivers, the provision of caregiver-friendly services as well as assisting in the setting up and facilitation of caregiver support groups.

Questions

Question 12.1	What does the term 'informal caregiver' mean to you and what are the differences between 'informal' and 'formal' carers?
Question 12.2	How would you assess the needs of a caregiver? What tools, if any, would you use? Who would you go to for advice? What would you assess?
Question 12.3	What four things could you do to support a caregiver within a GP practice or community healthcare centre?
Question 12.4	What four things could you do to support a caregiver within a hospital setting?
Question 12.5	How would you set up and facilitate a caregiver support group?

REFERENCES

Aldridge, H and Hughes, C. (2016) *Informal Carers and Poverty in the UK*. New Policy Institute. Available at: www.npi.org.uk/files/2114/6411/1359/Carers_and_poverty_in_the_UK_-_full_report.pdf (accessed 4 January 2022).

Carers Trust (2020) *Carers Trust Social Care Survey 2020*. Available at: https://carers.org/our-social-care-campaign/carers-trust-social-care-survey-2020 (accessed 4 January 2022).

Carers Trust (undated) *About Caring*. Available at: https://carers.org/about-caring/about-caring (accessed 4 January 2022).

Carers UK (2014) *Facts about Carers 2014*. Available from: www.carersuk.org/for-professionals/policy/policy-library/facts-about-carers-2014 (accessed 4 January 2022).

Carers UK (2019a) *State of Caring: A snapshot of unpaid care in the UK*. Available at: www.carersuk.org/images/News__campaigns/CUK_State_of_Caring_2019_Report.pdf (accessed 4 January 2022).

Carers UK (2019b) *Facts About Carers*. Available at: www.carersuk.org/images/Facts_about_Carers_2019.pdf (accessed 4 January 2022).

Carers UK (undated) *Fairer for Carers – background information*. Available at: www.carersuk.org/news-and-campaigns/campaigns/fairer-for-carers-background (accessed 4 January 2022).

Department of Health and Social Care (2018) *Carers action plan 2018–2020*. Available at: https://assets.publishing.service.gov.uk/government/uploads/system/uploads/attachment_data/file/713781/carers-action-plan-2018-2020.pdf (accessed 4 January 2022).

Foundation for People with Learning Disabilities (undated) *Learning disability statistics: effects of being a carer*. Available at: www.learningdisabilities.org.uk/learning-disabilities/help-information/Learning-Disability-Statistics-/187702 (accessed 4 January 2022).

Gressmann, M. (2014) Changing roles of family carers. *Learning Disability Practice*, **17(4)**: 34–9.

HM Government (2021) *The National Minimum Wage in 2021*. Available at: www.gov.uk/government/publications/the-national-minimum-wage-in-2021 (accessed 4 January 2022).

Ouldred, E. and Bryant, C. (2008) 'The older adult, intellectual impairments and the dementias'. In Clark, L. and Griffiths, P. (2008) *Learning Disability and Other Intellectual Impairments*. John Wiley & Sons.

RESOURCES

Carers Trust (2020) *Carers Trust Social Care Survey 2020*. Available at: https://carers.org/our-social-care-campaign/carers-trust-social-care-survey-2020 (accessed 4 January 2022).

Carers UK (2019) *Facts about Carers*. Available at: www.carersuk.org/images/Facts_about_Carers_2019.pdf (accessed 4 January 2022).

Carers UK *Fairer for carers*. Available at: www.carersuk.org/news-and-campaigns/campaigns/fairer-for-carers (accessed 4 January 2022).

Houses of Parliament website: www.parliament.uk/business/bills-and-legislation/ (accessed 4 January 2022).

For the Parliamentary Acts listed below (all accessed 4 January 2022):

- Carers (Recognition and Services) Act 1995: www.legislation.gov.uk/ukpga/1995/12/contents
- Carers and Disabled Children Act 2000: www.legislation.gov.uk/ukpga/2000/16/contents (this Act has now been repealed and much of it included in subsequent Parliamentary Acts. However, this Act may be of historical interest)
- Carers (Equal Opportunities) Act 2004: www.legislation.gov.uk/ukpga/2004/15/contents
- Equality Act 2010: www.legislation.gov.uk/ukpga/2010/15/contents
- Care Act 2014: www.legislation.gov.uk/ukpga/2014/23/contents

Policy paper: *Recognised, Valued and Supported: next steps for the carers strategy:* www.gov.uk/government/publications/recognised-valued-and-supported-next-steps-for-the-carers-strategy (accessed 4 January 2022).

Chapter 13
Disability and carer discrimination

AIMS AND LEARNING OUTCOMES

The aims of this chapter are to highlight:

- The existence of disability discrimination in the UK
- The meanings of discrimination and hate incidents and crimes
- Anti-discrimination legislation
- Those who experience learning disabilities, whether as service users, caregivers or care professionals, and their experiences of disability discrimination and hate incidents and crimes
- The roles of the nurse in tackling disability discrimination and hate incidents and crimes.

By the end of this chapter you will be able to:

- Discuss the meanings and definitions of discrimination and hate incidents and crimes and the relationship between the three
- Discuss the impact that disability discrimination as a hate incident or crime can have on those with a learning disability and their families
- Discuss your roles as a nurse and a citizen in tackling disability discrimination.

PAUSE FOR THOUGHT 13.1

Disability discrimination is a hate incident: discuss.

13.1 Introduction

It could be suggested that those with a learning disability have endured a very long history of discrimination on the grounds of their disability and societal responses to this disability. Such discrimination arguably begins prior to birth and, again arguably, lasts until after the person has died. Family members as caregivers are also likely to experience discrimination due to their association with the person with a learning disability (disability by proxy) (see *Chapter 12* for a more detailed exposition of examples of potential caregiver discrimination). In this, those with a learning disability are not alone as they are likely to share a common history of discrimination with those who have physical disability issues or mental health issues, come from a BAME background or culture or are LGBTQ+. These are the claims and issues that are central to this chapter.

13.2 What is discrimination?

It may be helpful here to understand what discrimination actually is before we go on to discuss how discrimination affects those with a learning disability.

To put it very simply, discrimination means to treat one person differently from another. However, there is much more to the term 'discrimination' than that! After all, I engage, interact and communicate with, and therefore treat my boss differently from the way I do my wife or my friends down at the pub. This is only right and proper as this involves both professional and personal boundaries. Is this discrimination though?

Discrimination could also be described as where one person is treated not so much differently but either better or worse than another person on the basis of certain characteristics. Discrimination can be divided into two forms: positive and negative. Positive discrimination is where one person is offered more favourable opportunities and conditions than another in order to allow the first person to engage and compete within certain aspects of society and socioeconomic life, such as employment and education. Positive discrimination allows for a 'level playing field' that permits all people to engage in socially valued activities. Making 'reasonable adjustments' for those who have disabilities or are caregivers could be argued to be a form of positive discrimination.

However, negative discrimination is:

"The act of denying rights, benefits, justice, equitable treatment, or access to facilities available to all others, to an individual or group of people because of their race, age, gender, handicap or other defining characteristic" (Megson, 2011).

Many people, because they are old, fat, thin, poor, wealthy, unemployed, disabled, black, Asian, or a single or teenage mum, can be discriminated against. Often, some people do not need a reason to discriminate. According to the Equality Act 2010, in terms of discrimination and employment, discrimination against a disabled employee occurs if, on the grounds of that employee's disability, the employee is treated less favourably than an employee not having that particular disability whose relevant circumstances are the same or not materially different from those of the disabled person.

Although using Wikipedia as a source of information may be frowned upon because some entries may be less than accurate, it is worth quoting in full its definition of discrimination:

"Discrimination is the act of making unjustified distinctions between human beings based on the groups, classes, or other categories to which they are perceived to belong. People may be discriminated on the basis of race, gender, age, religion, or sexual orientation, as well as other categories. Discrimination especially occurs when individuals or groups are unfairly treated in a way which is worse than other people are treated, on the basis of their actual or perceived membership in certain groups or social categories. It involves restricting members of one group from opportunities or privileges that are available to members of another group."

(http://en.wikipedia.org/wiki/Discrimination)

The Wikipedia definition is relatively straightforward in that discrimination is based on one person's or group's view and thus response to, and interaction with another person or group on the grounds of difference, whether perceived or real, and that such responses and interactions are often irrational. However, the last part of this definition suggests that although largely discredited, discriminatory practices still exist under various guises such as 'affirmative action'.

What then is the definition of 'hate crime', and are there any links between the meanings of disability discrimination and hate crimes?

The Metropolitan Police offer the following suggestions:

"In most crimes it is something the victim has in their possession or control that motivates the offender to commit the crime. With hate crime it is 'who' the victim is, or 'what' the victim appears to be that motivates the offender to commit the crime. A hate crime is defined as 'any criminal offence which is perceived by the victim or any other person, to be motivated by hostility or prejudice based on a person's race or perceived race; religion or perceived religion; sexual orientation or perceived sexual orientation; disability or perceived disability and any crime motivated by hostility or prejudice against a person who is transgender or perceived to be transgender."

Whilst discrimination may not necessarily involve a 'criminal element' and thus will not sit easily in the above definition of hate crime, discrimination may be viewed as a *hate incident*. A hate incident (Metropolitan Police, undated):

"… is any incident which the victim, or anyone else, thinks is based on someone's prejudice towards them because of their race, religion, sexual orientation, disability or because they are transgender."

Not all hate incidents will amount to criminal offences, but it is equally important that these are reported to and recorded by the police. Evidence of the hate element is not a requirement. The person does not need to personally perceive the incident to be hate-related. It would be enough if another person, a witness or even a police officer thought that the incident was hate-related.

Thus, disability discrimination can be viewed as a hate incident rather than a hate crime, although disability discrimination as a hate incident can lead to disability discrimination as a hate crime if the incident either breaks or leads to the breaking of criminal rather than civil law.

13.3 Anti-discrimination legislation

There have been three main pieces of anti-discrimination legislation that will affect those with a learning disability. It must be kept in mind that these Parliamentary Acts highlight disability discrimination in general and are not learning disability specific, there being no learning disability specific law (the Autism Act 2009 deals specifically with autism and not with learning disability):

- The Disability Discrimination Act (DDA) 1995
- The Human Rights Act 1997
- The Equality Act 2010

Each of these three Parliamentary Acts will be briefly explored below.

13.3.1 Disability Discrimination Act 1995

November 2020 marked 25 years since the Disability Discrimination Act became law in the UK. The law was the first of its kind to protect those with disabilities from discrimination in areas including employment, the provision of goods and services, education and transport. It was replaced by the Equality Act 2010, which kept many of the same provisions as the original Act.

The Act was passed by the then Prime Minister John Major's Conservative Government and came into force in 1995. While the Race Relations Act 1976 and the Sex Discrimination Act 1975 provided legal protection from discrimination on grounds of race and gender, those with a disability lacked similar protection enshrined in law. It could be argued, however, that racial and gender / sexual discrimination still exist today despite these two pieces of legislation.

In the early 1990s, thousands of protesters, including many disabled people, took to the streets demanding new legislation. These protesters included the Disabled People's Direct Action Network (DAN). Protests escalated as the 1990s progressed, with DAN moving from marches and demonstrations to more radical action, including protesters handcuffing themselves to buses.

The Disability Discrimination Act 1995 defined disability as a physical or mental impairment which has a substantial and long-term adverse effect on a person's ability to carry out normal day-to-day activities.

The Act provided protection against discrimination in several areas, including:

- employment and occupation;
- education;
- transport;
- the provision of goods; and
- the exercise of public functions.

The Act was the first of its kind to protect disabled people from multiple kinds of discrimination. These included:

- direct discrimination: where a disabled person is treated less favourably than another person due to their disability;

- failure to make a reasonable adjustment: where any workplace practice or feature of the premises puts a disabled worker at a disadvantage; and
- victimisation: where a person is treated unfavourably because they made a complaint about their treatment as a disabled person.

13.3.2 Human Rights Act 1998

The Human Rights Act gives effect to the human rights set out in the European Convention on Human Rights. These rights are called Convention rights.

Examples of Convention or human rights include:
- the right to life
- the right to respect for private and family life
- the right to freedom of religion and belief.

The Human Rights Act protects everyone in the UK, regardless of who they are. Those who believe that their rights have been breached can seek the remedy of the courts. Thus, if a person believes that they are being discriminated against in the areas of forming sexual relationships or told that they are not allowed to have children (the right to respect for private and family life) on the grounds of having a learning disability for example, they can take their case to court.

13.3.3 Equality Act 2010

The Disability Discrimination Act 1995 was replaced in England, Scotland and Wales by the Equality Act 2010. The Disability Discrimination Act remains on the statute book in Northern Ireland. Many amendments to anti-discrimination legislation that have been made in the rest of the UK have been introduced in Northern Ireland through secondary legislation. However, some groups have called for a simplification of the legislation in Northern Ireland to bring equality legislation in line with the rest of the UK.

Under the Equality Act 2010, disability is one of nine protected characteristics. According to the provisions of the Act, those with disabilities continue to be protected from direct and indirect discrimination, harassment related to disability, and victimisation. Much of the original text of the 1995 Act was directly incorporated into the 2010 Act.

13.4 Experiences of those who have a learning disability

"It all started with shouting names and stealing my things. Over the years it's got more serious. I get nervous, shake and have panic attacks.

I'm Kelly and I've been a victim of hate crime. At first the bullies at school used to call me names because I wasn't as fast as other kids at learning things. Once I went to the park with my brother and they stole my walkman and cassettes from me.

It got worse and worse from that day. Now I'm 41 and I still get called nasty names, now it's on the street. I try to walk straight down the road, try not to listen to what they are shouting. They follow me home, ring my bell, wake me up and bang on my door.

It causes me stress and makes my blood pressure high. I just want them to stop, it's not fair.

When I tell the police they just say: 'Walk away Kelly,' or 'just ignore them Kelly.' But I want it to change. I want people to be nicer to me. That's why I want to tell the government, because this is serious."

(*Kelly and Sue's story*: Mencap, undated (a))

Discrimination is not limited to people with disabilities, as people who are lesbian, gay, bisexual or transgender, from a different cultural or ethnic background or those who experience mental health problems have had to endure decades of discrimination. Anyone who looks or sounds different in any way from 'the norm' appears to be fair game as can be illustrated in *Kelly and Sue's story* that is presented by Mencap (see above). Verbal bullying and harassment of those with a learning disability appears to be a common feature in some people's lives.

However, with the increase of internet bullying and discrimination has also come an increase in victims of such bullying and discrimination engaging in acts of self-harm and even suicide. It is not just those with disabilities who are likely to be subject to negative discrimination with often tragic results.

A number of newspaper articles spanning the past 15 years appears to confirm the often painful nature of actual or perceived discrimination. The first concerns a mother who kills her 12-year-old autistic son by throwing him off the Humber Bridge and then takes her own life by following him (Wainwright, 2006). The second concerns a young man with a learning disability who was bullied and made to carry out absolutely horrendous acts by those whom he thought were his friends. These so-called friends eventually murdered him (Williams, 2010). Williams reports on an incident of 'mate crime' and it may be worth reading Mencap (undated (b)) for a brief exploration of this term. A local politician in Cornwall, Collin Brewer (Mail Online, 2013) stated that children with a disability are like deformed lambs and should be killed by throwing them against a brick wall. He believed that the money that would be saved through the killing of disabled children would open and run ten public toilets. A fourth such article can be found in the Guardian online (www.theguardian.com/commentisfree/2014/apr/15/hard-life-disabled-hating-bigot-mayor). A one-time Conservative councillor and mayor of Swindon, Nick Martin, aged 63, was found guilty of breaching the members' code of conduct after Labour complained about comments that he made. Labour councillors said they heard him say: "Are we still letting Mongols [people with Down's syndrome] have sex with each other?"

Although Brewer and Martin were not only "last year's" but "last decade's" news, anecdotally many people with a learning disability and/or autism do not believe that Brewer and Martin were alone in believing that those with a learning disability are 'trash' and that as a society we have not moved on since then. Most of those who are victims of hate incidents and crimes share that they are still mentally and emotionally scarred by their experiences. Many of these are still too afraid to even leave their homes for fear of what might happen to them. Disability discrimination, whether or not such discrimination can be seen as a 'hate incident', can cause symptoms in some people that are pretty close to post-traumatic stress disorder.

Anecdotal evidence seems to suggest that many people with a learning disability still experience poor or non-existent care and support services, and support by care staff who do not seem to care and cannot be bothered and do not want to know. Such poor services and care can be seen as a form of disability discrimination. A Mencap report in 2013 (Mencap, 2013a) highlights the scale of discrimination faced by people with a learning disability in NHS settings following the publication of findings from an independent enquiry into the deaths of those with a learning disability. Systemic failings in most if not all aspects of healthcare were highlighted in this report. Whilst such discrimination may be explained at least in part by a lack of knowledge and understanding about those with a learning disability, their health and care needs and forms of communication, not all discrimination can be so justified. An inherent uncritical acceptance of societal attitudes regarding the 'value' of those with a learning disability must also play a large part.

In another Mencap report (Mencap, 2013b) it is suggested that whilst in the two years from 2011/12 to 2012/13 there were 124 000 disability hate crimes being reported to the police, only 1% of these resulted in prosecutions. This seems to relay the message that disability hate incidents and hate crime are very low down on the priorities of police forces and the legal system.

More recent information and discussions around the range of discrimination that those with a learning disability often face can be found at EHRC (2020), BIHR (2016), NHS England (2019) and Mencap (undated (c)). These seem to indicate that disability discrimination, far from diminishing or coming to an end, is still prevalent and is likely to be so for the foreseeable future.

It could be argued that such a low level of priority, a low level stemming from ignorance, is widespread even if covert. On the level of society, disability discrimination makes us all poorer. It brutalises and dehumanises us, as can be seen by Brewer's and Martin's comments. Discrimination engenders and perpetuates discrimination and with that, the willingness to diminish and ultimately destroy those who are in any way different.

Whilst the more contemporaneous evidence cited above may not mention specific incidents or people who discriminate along similar lines to Brewer, it is not beyond the realms of possibility that disability discrimination can move through hate incidence to hate crime and even further to programmes of eugenics, where only the 'non-disabled' would be allowed to live. While some people may view this as extreme and an exercise in hyperbole, others, mainly those with disabilities, are fearful that such an extreme scenario could happen, with politicians such as Brewer and Martin being the tip of an iceberg.

It could further be argued that disability discrimination affects care professionals and those discriminated against, as well as society. It is not being suggested here that the vast majority of nurses and other healthcare professionals deliberately discriminate against those with a learning disability, although it has to be said that a tiny minority do. Disability discrimination is likely to be very subtle and unconscious, possibly reflecting a 'culture of discrimination' such as that highlighted in the Report of the Mid Staffordshire NHS Foundation Trust Public Inquiry, also known as the Francis Report (TSO, 2013). Nurses may be unaware that they are engaging in disability-focused discriminatory behaviour.

Again, BIHR (2016), NHS England (2019) and various Mencap reports all suggest that disability discrimination is still experienced by those with a learning disability and that cultures that at the very least allow for disability discrimination still prevail in some areas of health and social care and in the criminal justice system.

Disability discrimination demeans, brutalises, impoverishes and dehumanises care professionals and can often lead to stress and burnout and the possibility of abuse. Disability discrimination, indeed any form of discrimination, could lead to the nurse being in breach of the Nursing and Midwifery Council's code of professional conduct (NMC, 2018) and this would therefore be grounds for professional misconduct charges. In relation to those with disabilities, as has already been mentioned, discrimination leads to rejection, humiliation, fear, intimidation, isolation, loneliness, anger and even in extreme cases the destruction and extinction of the person. One has only to explore the thinking and rationalisation behind the behaviour exhibited by care staff at Winterbourne View (NHS England, 2014), Whorlton Hall (BBC, 2019) and Cawston Park hospital (Setchell, 2021) (all privately run by 'for profit' companies) to see concrete examples of the outcome of disability discrimination. It is extremely unlikely that these will be the last incidents of discriminatory hate crimes that will be seen.

PAUSE FOR THOUGHT 13.2

The central question here is: what kind of society, what kind of world are we living in that turns its back on such abuse and discrimination and allows it to happen? Is this the kind of society that we want for ourselves and our children?

13.5 The roles of the nurse

Disability discrimination, be it covert, subconscious or deliberate, is real, it happens and it often has profound effects on people. The question is: what can nurses do to challenge such discrimination? The following may be useful starting points:

- Nurses need to be aware of their own personal biases, prejudices, beliefs, social attitudes and world views. Nurses are only human and are not machines and will, whether they like it or not, have their own prejudices, beliefs and attitudes, many of which may reflect the prejudices of society at large. The trick is to acknowledge them and how they can impact upon the care and support services that nurses offer. Following on from that, nurses need to be aware of and reflect upon the biases, beliefs, prejudices and attitudes in others and how these impact upon the lives of those around them. Nurses also need to be aware of the personal and societal attitudes and beliefs of those who worked at places like Winterbourne View and Whorlton Hall and that led to the horrendous treatment of those living at these places. If nurses are not aware of and do not understand these attitudes and beliefs, they run the risk of being condemned to not only holding these same views and prejudices but acting upon them.

- Care professionals need to be aware of, understand and implement organisational policies on anti-discrimination. At the very least healthcare professionals must be aware of where these policies and procedures are kept and have read many of them during their induction period. Policies on anti-discriminatory behaviour should form a crucial aspect of these policies.
- It would also be expected that nurses and other healthcare professionals are fully aware of and understand both the contents and the underlying philosophy of the relevant anti-discrimination legislation and how this legislation seeks to tackle discrimination in all its forms.
- Active participation in professional development opportunities such as short courses and workshops, discussions with colleagues and research can be excellent ways of raising knowledge around discriminatory issues.
- If you do engage in behaviour that discriminates, be willing and prepared to justify your attitudes and behaviours and accept their consequences. You must also be prepared and willing to challenge discriminatory practice both in yourself and in others. Nurses are governed by the Nursing and Midwifery Council's code of professional conduct. Read, understand and abide by this code.
- Finally, it is recommended that whatever you do, record and report any forms of discrimination that you encounter, its causes and effects on the individual patient or service user, what could have been done differently and what was done to challenge the discrimination and its outcomes.

13.6 Conclusion

Discrimination of those with various disabilities on the grounds of their disability has been a 'fixture' in many people's lives for decades, if not centuries. Whilst disability discrimination in many areas of life is now illegal under the 2010 Equalities Act, those with a learning disability still experience discrimination. As a nurse, you have a primary duty to do no harm. This duty must include recognising and challenging disability discrimination, whether such discrimination manifests itself in beliefs, attitudes, words or actions, wherever and whenever it is found. Not to do so results in colluding in such discrimination. Always remember, disability discrimination, whatever form it takes, is a hate incident, an incident which has the potential to lead to a hate crime, and must be challenged as such.

CHAPTER SUMMARY

Key points to take away from *Chapter 13*:
- ☑ Discrimination involves the act of treating people differently and often leads to the denying of rights, benefits, justice, equitable treatment, or access to facilities available to all others, to an individual or group of people because of their race, age, gender, disability or other defining characteristic.
- ☑ Disability discrimination, although illegal, still continues in many environments and by many people including care staff (e.g. Winterbourne View and Whorlton Hall) and politicians.
- ☑ Disability discrimination can be seen as a hate incident which can cause severe psychological and emotional harm to the victim.
- ☑ The role of the nurse includes being aware of and understanding personal beliefs and attitudes to those with a learning disability, being aware of and understanding employer policies and anti-discrimination legislation, and challenging discrimination when and where it occurs.

Questions

Question 13.1   How would you define disability discrimination?

Question 13.2   Is disability discrimination a hate crime, a hate incident or both? Justify your answer.

Question 13.3   Which forms of discrimination could those with a learning disability experience? (You may find the following website useful here: www.brighton-hove.gov.uk/content/council-and-democracy/equality/disability-hate-incidents)

Question 13.4   Re-read the section above on experiences. What four steps can you take to challenge such discrimination?

Question 13.5   Reflect on your own beliefs regarding those with a learning disability. If you feel that your beliefs could be seen as being potentially discriminatory, what four steps can you take to challenge and change these beliefs?

REFERENCES

BBC (2019) Whorlton Hall: Hospital 'abused' vulnerable adults. Available at: www.bbc.co.uk/news/health-48367071 (accessed 4 January 2022).

British Institute of Human Rights (2016) *Learning disabilities and human rights: a practitioner's guide.* Available at: https://knowyourhumanrights.co.uk/resources/BIHR_Mental_Health_Practitioner_Resource_LearningDisability.pdf (accessed 4 January 2022).

Equality and Human Rights Commission (2020) *Disability discrimination.* Available at: www.equalityhumanrights.com/en/advice-and-guidance/disability-discrimination (accessed 4 January 2022).

Mail Online (2013) Collin Brewer resigns. Available at: www.dailymail.co.uk/news/article-2285773/Collin-Brewer-resigns-saying-Disabled-children-cost-down.html (accessed 4 January 2022).

Megson, D. (2011) Discrimination against disabilities: a life worth less? *British Journal of Healthcare Assistants*, **5(10)**: 495–8.

Mencap (2013a) *Mencap research: "scandal of avoidable death" as 1,200 people with a learning disability die needlessly every year in NHS care.* Available at: www.mencap.org.uk/press-release/mencap-research-scandal-avoidable-death-1200-people-learning-disability-die (accessed 4 January 2022).

Mencap (2013b) *Hear my voice: hate crime.* Available at: www.mencap.org.uk/get-involved/campaign-mencap/hear-my-voice/hear-my-voice-hate-crime (accessed 4 January 2022).

Mencap (undated (a)) *Kelly and Sue's story.* Available at: www.mencap.org.uk/get-involved/campaign-mencap/hear-my-voice/hear-my-voice-hate-crime (accessed 4 January 2022).

Mencap (undated (b)) *Mate and hate crime.* Available at: www.mencap.org.uk/advice-and-support/bullying-and-discrimination/mate-and-hate-crime (accessed 4 January 2022).

Mencap (undated (c)) *Stigma and discrimination – research and statistics.* Available at: www.mencap.org.uk/learning-disability-explained/research-and-statistics/stigma-and-discrimination-research-and (accessed 4 January 2022).

Metropolitan Police (undated) *What is hate crime?* Available at: www.met.police.uk/advice/advice-and-information/hco/hate-crime/what-is-hate-crime/ (accessed 4 January 2022).

NHS England (2014) *Winterbourne View – time for change.* Available at: www.england.nhs.uk/wp-content/uploads/2014/11/transforming-commissioning-services.pdf (accessed 4 January 2022).

NHS England (2019) *People with a learning disability, autism or both.* Available at: www.england.nhs.uk/wp-content/uploads/2020/01/Learning-disability-and-autism.pdf (accessed 4 January 2022).

Nursing and Midwifery Council (2018) *The Code: Professional standards of practice and behaviour for nurses, midwives and nursing associates.* NMC. Available at: www.nmc.org.uk/standards/code/ (accessed 4 January 2022).

Setchell, R. (2021) Cawston Park: Damning report into deaths of three people at Norfolk hospital. Available at: www.itv.com/news/anglia/2021-09-09/cawston-park-damning-report-into-deaths-of-three-people-at-norfolk-hospital (accessed 4 January 2022).

The Stationery Office (2013) *Report of the Mid Staffordshire NHS Foundation Trust Public Inquiry.* Executive summary available at: https://assets.publishing.service.gov.uk/government/uploads/system/uploads/attachment_data/file/279124/0947.pdf (accessed 4 January 2022).

Wainwright, M. (2006) A mother and son smiling at the station. Then two specks on the edge of a bridge. *The Guardian*. Available at: www.theguardian.com/uk/2006/apr/19/martinwainwright.mainsection (accessed 4 January 2022).

Williams, R. (2010) 'Mate crime' fears for people with learning disabilities. *The Guardian*. Available at: www.theguardian.com/society/2010/sep/14/learning-disabilities-mate-crime (accessed 4 January 2022).

RESOURCES

Care Act 2014: www.legislation.gov.uk/ukpga/2014/23/contents (accessed 4 January 2022).

Disability Discrimination Act 1995: www.legislation.gov.uk/ukpga/1995/50/contents (accessed 4 January 2022).

Equality Act 2010: www.legislation.gov.uk/ukpga/2010/15/contents (accessed 4 January 2022).

Human Rights Act 1998: www.legislation.gov.uk/ukpga/1998/42/contents (accessed 4 January 2022).

Chapter 14
Learning disability and spirituality

AIMS AND LEARNING OUTCOMES

The aims of this chapter are to highlight:

- The meaning of spirituality and the differences and similarities between spirituality and religion

- The barriers that prevent those with a learning disability from experiencing and expressing their spirituality

- The resources that are available that may assist those with a learning disability in experiencing and expressing their spiritual dimension

- How nurses can support those with a learning disability to experience and express their spirituality.

By the end of this chapter, you will be able to discuss with colleagues:

- The meaning of spirituality

- How spirituality is both similar to and different from religion

- The various barriers that could hinder or prevent those with a learning disability from engaging in and expressing their own spiritual identity

- The various resources that are available that could assist in a meaningful spiritual engagement, expression and identity

- How you as a nurse can assist those with a learning disability to so engage with, experience and express their spiritual identity by drawing up a five-point action plan.

14.1 Introduction

Much of this book has focused on perhaps the more physical aspects of working with and providing care and support for those with a learning disability. However, nurses must work within a holistic person-centred framework; they must plan, provide and assess and evaluate holistically and with the individual service user at its centre. Spirituality is a vital component of such holistic person-centred care.

Spirituality is often appended to end of life care as very much an 'afterthought'. Even then it may not be with a great deal of understanding of the needs of the person or comprehension that spirituality is for the whole of life and not just at the end of that life. Swinton (2002) argued that the spirituality of people with learning disabilities is under-researched and frequently misunderstood. Barber (2013) argued that those with a learning disability have as great a spiritual need and as much right to have that need met as anyone else in society. This is the central argument in this chapter.

I am indebted here to the *British Journal of Healthcare Assistants* for their very kind permission in allowing the use of definitions, meanings and barriers as they had been used in a series of articles written by me on spirituality for the *BJHCA*.

14.2 What is spirituality?

PAUSE FOR THOUGHT 14.1

Are you aware of, and comfortable with your own sense of the spiritual, with your own spiritual identity? Do you know what spirituality is and the similarities and differences between spirituality and religion?

What, then, is this thing called spirituality?
- Is it a thing or is it much more intimate and profound than that?
- How does spirituality manifest itself?
- Given that there may be some confusion between religion and spirituality, with these two concepts or phenomena appearing to mean the same thing, is spirituality the same as religion?
- What are its similarities with and differences to religion?
- In today's world, is spirituality relevant?
- Do I have the time, the ability, the skills and the resources to engage in another person's spirituality?

These and a hundred other questions spring to mind at the mere mention of spirituality.

Spirituality is a remarkably difficult concept to define and understand (Wattis, Curran and Rogers, 2017) and there are likely to be as many definitions of spirituality as there are people holding and professing such definitions or meanings. Spirituality is a broad concept with room for many perspectives and there are a wide range of meanings that can be given to the phenomenon of spirituality (Gardner, 2011; Bogdashina, 2013). MacKinlay (2006, p. 13) suggests that:

> *"Spirituality is the personal quest for understanding answers to ultimate questions about life, about meaning and about relationships to the sacred or the transcendent which may (or may not) lead to or arise from the development of religious rituals."*

MacKinlay (2006, p. 13) also suggests that spirituality refers to an ultimate meaning of self and life that is mediated through relationships with others and with God (however one defines this term), the environment, the arts and through religion.

In a survey of definitions of spirituality conducted and explored by McSherry (2007), the following were highlighted:

- Spirituality is my inner being. It is who I am. It is me expressed through my body, my thinking and my feelings (Stoll, 1989, p. 61)
- A quality that goes beyond religious affiliation, that strives for inspiration, reverence, awe, meaning and purpose. Spirituality can also be seen as a belief in a supernatural or divine force that has power over the universe and commands worship and obedience (Murray and Zentner, 1989, pp. 257 and 259)
- The way in which men and women may understand their existence and the action which comes from this understanding (Males and Boswell, 1990, p. 35)
- Spirituality refers to the propensity to make meaning through a sense of relatedness to dimensions that transcend the self in such a way that empowers and does not devalue the individual (Reed, 1992, p. 350)
- Spirituality is a personal search for meaning and purpose in life which may or may not be related to religion. It entails connection to self-chosen and/or religious beliefs, values and practices that gives meaning to life (Tanyi, 2002, p. 506).

Again, Wiseman (2006, p. 4) follows Schneiders (1989) in suggesting that spirituality has three interrelated dimensions or references:

- Spirituality is a fundamental aspect of the human being and what it means to be human
- Spirituality is the lived experience that actualises this fundamental aspect of humanness
- Spirituality is the study of this lived experience.

However, it could be suggested that spirituality is different from religion, although many people confuse the two and consider religion and spirituality as the same thing. So, what is religion?

MacKinlay (2006, p. 13) suggests that religion is:

"an organised system of beliefs, practices, rituals and symbols that is designed to facilitate closeness to the sacred or transcendent through fostering an understanding of one's relationship and responsibility to others in living together in a community. Religion is part of spirituality. The practice of religion is a way that humans relate to the sacred and to others".

Murray and Zentner (1989, p. 259) suggest that religion is:

"a system of beliefs, a comprehensive code of ethics or philosophy, a set of practices that are followed, a church affiliation, the conscious pursuit of any object the person holds as supreme".

Thus, spirituality could be seen as one way that an individual understands and connects to oneself, others, the world and the 'divine' (however one defines the divine), whilst religion provides a community and a structure that nurtures and provides a framework for this understanding and connectivity to take root and grow.

14.3 Barriers to experiencing and practising spirituality

Those with a learning disability have the same right as anyone else to experience and express their own spiritual identity and to do so in ways that they feel comfortable with. However, it could be suggested that those with a learning disability face and experience barriers to such spiritual experiences and expression in much the same way that they do in other areas of life, as a result of having a learning disability.

What, then, are these barriers? Those with a learning disability could experience some, perhaps many, of the following:

- Spiritual and faith community support being a 'curate's egg', i.e. good in parts. Where it is good, it is very good and where it is bad it is bad!
- Those with learning disabilities are often ignored, patronised and treated as little children, regardless of whether the person is an adult with adult needs and life experiences
- Those with a learning disability are often lumped together as a homogenous group instead of being engaged with as an individual, and without taking into account the background, culture, abilities and wishes of individual service users (one size fits all!)
- Faith leaders and faith communities tend not to understand either learning disability as a concept or those with a learning disability.

Little genuine and sensitive help is offered, either by faith communities or health and social care staff, to support those with a learning disability to be comfortable with and express their own spirituality.

Resulting from a number of informal conversations with those with a learning disability, a number of anecdotal comments were made regarding experiences of spirituality:

- "My priest does not understand me"
- "The care staff where I live are too busy to make time to really be with me, to listen to me"
- "The care staff where I live are embarrassed when I try to pray"
- "The care staff where I live seem to find my attempts at prayer funny"
- "I feel trapped in a system that does not care"
- "Too much noise, too much busyness"
- "I have no contact with my local mosque" (the same could apply equally to other faith communities)
- "I am a Jew, but the only religious service that I can go to is run by the hospital-based Church of England vicar"
- "I often feel ignored by my church"
- "I feel that I am being treated as a little child"
- "I feel lonely. Everyone talks to each other, but no one talks or listens to me"
- "No one helps me to talk to God".

It could be that some of these barriers result from a lack of understanding of those with a learning disability by faith communities and their leaders, while others result from issues within the care environment.

Again, those with a learning disability may have been viewed as:

- unable to engage in spirituality in any meaningful way, due to assumptions about their lack of ability to understand and reason (Gaventa, 2010)
- 'holy and saintly simple people', as God's 'specially chosen'. As a result of this, those with a learning disability were often put on pedestals, adulated and out of the reach of 'ordinary' people
- the result of sin, either their own or, more likely, their parents' or grandparents' (see St. John's Gospel 9:2 for an example of this from the Christian tradition). This, again, has a similar 'outsider' effect. It was a popular idea and doctrine at the time the Christian Gospels were written and compiled, and in the Jewish faith and early Christian church, that all suffering, illness and disability in this life had their origins in sin, hence the suggestion in Jn 9:2 that the man was born blind as a result of his own or his parents' sin. This position has been discredited by biblical scholars for at least 50 years, although there may be certain parts of the Christian tradition who would continue to uphold this interpretation.

As a further result, those with a learning disability became outsiders.

All of these were likely to have a negative impact upon a spiritual identity that those with a learning disability could meaningfully own, experience and express.

14.4 Spiritual resources

Having briefly highlighted a number of potential barriers that could impact upon and potentially prevent a person with a learning disability from meaningfully owning, experiencing and expressing their own authentic spirituality, the following range of resources (a range that is by no means exhaustive) may be useful; some of these resources may be more helpful to those with a learning disability than to nurses, whilst others may be more useful to nurses than to those with a learning disability.

14.4.1 Hospital chaplains

The hospital chaplaincy team are employed to provide spiritual and faith support to patients, service users, staff and patients' families. However, chaplains who have been appropriately trained in providing spiritual and faith community support to those with a learning disability provide a different form of support to such patients during their stay in hospital than many if not most nurses. Key roles of the chaplaincy team and individual chaplains are to provide a link for the patient and staff between the hospital ward or clinical setting and the wide variety of faith communities, and to be a listening friend to patients and staff alike. They are also involved in the ongoing professional development of hospital staff regarding dignity, spirituality and faith communities. These teams can be contacted via the hospital switchboard and/or hospital chapel or multi-faith centre. The website for the College of Health Care Chaplains is www.healthcarechaplains.org.

14.4.2 Hospital guidelines and policies

Treating patients and service users with respect and dignity will form the cornerstone of most, if not all hospital, NHS Trust or other health and social care providers' policies and procedures. This will include policies on respecting the religious, faith and spiritual beliefs of all patients, service users and staff as well as equality, diversity and inclusion. It is likely that, during a new employee's induction period, they will either be given a complete set of these policies or be encouraged to locate and read these policies and will be expected to sign to say that they have read them. It is always good practice for established and experienced staff to similarly locate and read these policies, many of which will be updated over time.

14.4.3 Local faith communities

Those with a learning disability have as much right to attend and participate in the spiritual, liturgical, pastoral and social life of their preferred faith community as anyone else. Whilst most general acute hospitals will have a multi-faith chaplaincy team who will support patients and service users who have a learning disability, it would still be useful to forge links with the person's own faith community. This is so that such faith communities could maintain contact with the person whilst they are in hospital and ensure that the person with a learning disability is still included in the spiritual, liturgical and pastoral life of their faith community. This is particularly important if the person with a learning disability is likely to be in hospital for any length of time.

14.4.4 Jean Vanier and L'Arche

Vanier was a French–Canadian philosopher, theologian, prolific writer and humanitarian who, in 1964, invited two people who had learning disabilities to live with him in a small village in France. Out of this small and simple beginning grew L'Arche, an international network of small community homes for those with learning disabilities run on largely Christian lines. Vanier has been disgraced over recent years as a result of him engaging in the sexual abuse of women (something that L'Arche has never condoned or tried to hide), but L'Arche itself has continued to thrive and has perhaps grown stronger as a result of the way that it has dealt with the scandal caused by Vanier. There are eight L'Arche communities in England (London, Ipswich, Preston, Manchester, Dover, Bognor, Nottingham and Liverpool) most of which are based around community homes, two in Scotland (Edinburgh and Inverness) and one in Wales (Brecon) – see www.larche.org.uk. Alongside these communities exist 'faith and light' ecumenical faith groups where those with learning disabilities and their friends and families come together to explore and engage in the spiritual dimension of the human journey (www.faithandlight.org.uk).

14.4.5 Mindfulness

The Buddhist-based practice of mindfulness exercises on which mindfulness-based cognitive therapy (MBCT) is loosely based, is a way of paying attention to the present moment, using spiritual methods such as meditation, breathing and yoga (www.mentalhealth.org.uk/a-to-z/m/mindfulness). Mindfulness training, as a way of reducing stress, helps us become more aware of our thoughts and feelings so that instead of being overwhelmed by them, we are better able to manage them. In perhaps more practical terms, mindfulness is a way of being slowly and quietly but totally present and connected to the present moment and to the totality (mind, body and spirit) of both the self and other people within this moment in time.

14.4.6 John Swinton and Kairos

The Kairos Forum was established by John Swinton (professor of practical theology at the University of Aberdeen) and Cristina Gangemi, to provide advice, information, advocacy, and support for individuals who have a learning disability and their families regarding spirituality, religious practice and the vital role that those with a learning disability and their families have within communities. The creation of a space for the development of networks of lay people, professionals and religious communities was seen as crucial as a way of providing information regarding spirituality and learning disability (www.kairosforum.org).

14.4.7 Books and journal articles

There is a vast library of books, academic papers and conference presentations that explores the rich and varied meanings and lived experiences of spirituality, both as part of and outside of faith communities; too many to highlight here. There is also an increasing number of books and nursing journal articles / papers as well as conference presentations that focus on spirituality, religious faith and healthcare, as can be seen in the references given below. Many of these explore spirituality and faith community engagement of those who have a learning disability. These books and articles are well worth exploring further.

14.4.8 Slow nursing

Many nurses work in a highly pressurised and fast-paced hospital or clinical setting, where timeliness and accuracy are of paramount importance. Days are carefully scheduled with treatments, tests and nursing care. 'Slow nursing', which originated in the USA, is more of a slow-moving, 'sit-on-the-bed-and-talk' kind of nursing. It takes time to get to know the patients and their worries, problems and hopes, to gain their trust and to support them. Patients and service users with a learning disability must feel comfortable with the nurse, must be able to trust them before allowing that nurse to work with them. This building up of a culture of mutual trust and confidence is likely to be a vital aspect of spiritual connectedness.

14.5 The role of the nurse

As a nurse, you have a professional responsibility to take into account and accommodate the spiritual beliefs and practices of patients and service users – including those with learning disabilities – during the provision of care, and to safeguard the right to hold and express such beliefs. This holds true regardless of where you work. However, the person—and never forget that they are a person and not just a patient, not just a set of health conditions—may be in your care for a few days, a week or two or a couple of months. Whilst you may not have the luxury of having the time to get to know the person well, you must make every encounter count.

First of all, it is vital that you are aware of the importance of recording in the person's care notes that the person wishes to explore and experience their spiritual identity and the steps that you should take to help facilitate this. Such information is likely to be important to yourself and your colleagues and helps with the continuity of nursing care.

Secondly, it is vital that you are aware of, comfortable with and understand your own spiritual and religious identity and journey. Without such awareness and understanding, it may be difficult to engage with the spiritual and religious identity and journey of another (Barber, 2013). Allow the patient or service user to gently guide you and take the lead in their own spiritual dance. Always give those with a learning disability space to share—and care professionals the space to listen and understand (Swinton, 2001). It may be helpful to compile a calendar of major spiritual and religious festivals and understand the spiritual significance of these festivals in the lives of people. Such calendars can be easily obtained from:

- the internet
- some diaries (although the information is likely to be incomplete and may highlight religious festivals and dates for a very small number of religions)
- local social services
- hospital chaplaincy services
- hospital-based equality and diversity champions.

Trying to settle on a workable definition of spirituality that most people can 'buy into' is very difficult and complex, as can be seen from the discussion in the previous section, and this difficulty can also apply to assessing spiritual needs, be the assessment 'formal' or 'informal'. The ongoing assessment of a person's spirituality is likely to be key to any support that may be offered. There are a range of tools available that may be useful in assessing a person's spiritual identity and needs. However, these assessment tools (see below) are very dated and do not explore the spirituality of those with a learning disability, issues that are likely to affect their validity and value. Therefore, these assessment tools must be used with caution and may need to be adapted to meet the spiritual needs of those with a learning disability. Organisations that focus on spirituality and learning disability such as the Kairos Forum, Faith and Light, and Through the Roof (www.throughtheroof.org/) may be useful in that regard.

- Multi-dimensional Religiosity scales (King and Hunt, 1972)
- The Spiritual Assessment Inventory (Hall and Edwards, 2002)
- The Spiritual Needs Assessment for Patients (SNAP) (Sharma *et al.*, 2012)
- Spiritual Care Needs Inventory (SCNI) (Wu *et al.*, 2016)
- FICA (Puchalski and Romer, 2000)
- F.A.I.T.H (King, 2002)
- Spiritual History Scale in Four Dimensions (Hays *et al.*, 2001).

Whilst the age of many of these assessments may affect their validity and value, the underlying ideas may still be valid and could form the basis of a new 'purpose-designed' assessment tool that is valid, relevant and fit for purpose, being designed around the spiritual needs of those with a learning disability. The learning disability liaison nurse and the multi-faith chaplaincy team are likely to be very useful when seeking advice and guidance regarding a wide range of spiritual and religious beliefs and practices which could then be adapted to meet the needs of those with a learning disability.

Those with severe or profound and multiple learning disabilities may experience major communication difficulties. This can lead to difficulties in expressing beliefs, needs, preferences or participating in activities that are considered part of the social, cultural and spiritual life of a particular faith community. Therefore, take time to really communicate and listen to your patients and service users. The use of photographs or simple pictures denoting religious beliefs and spiritual and socio-cultural activities may be helpful, as might resources such as 'books beyond words' (books comprising simple pictures that tell a story without the use of words). *Going to Church*, co-authored by Professor John Swinton from Aberdeen University, will be particularly useful here (https://booksbeyondwords.co.uk/bookshop/going-to-church) and could be adapted to meet the spiritual needs of those who do not identify themselves as Christian.

Some belief systems attach particular importance to personal hygiene before prayer, with hygiene being intimately linked to concepts of inner cleanliness and purity. Those who possess such beliefs and have a learning disability may need more regular assistance with washing whilst on the ward or in the care home. Ensure that facilities and privacy around personal hygiene as an aspect of spiritual or religious / liturgical activity are available to assist those with a learning disability, should they require it.

At all times, privacy is crucial and is to be respected and maintained. As well as being understood in terms of the right to privacy, access to personal space and time alone is an important aspect of allowing individuals to develop their understanding of their world, reflect on their circumstances and beliefs, pray or otherwise contemplate their environment and how they relate to and engage with it. Conversely, engagement with others may also be an important aspect of a person's spirituality and such engagement can be facilitated through the communal celebration of major religious feasts and festivals as well as access to the person's faith community.

It would be helpful although not always easy to work mindfully. Professor Mark Williams, former director of the Oxford Mindfulness Centre, says that mindfulness means knowing directly what is going on inside and outside ourselves, moment by moment.

> *"An important part of mindfulness is reconnecting with our bodies and the sensations they experience. This means waking up to the sights, sounds, smells and tastes of the present moment. That might be something as simple as the feel of a banister as we walk upstairs. Another important part of mindfulness is an awareness of our thoughts and feelings as they happen moment to moment."* (Williams, as cited on NHS, 2018)

Through mindfulness, we become centred in the here and now, becoming totally aware of what is happening around us and, more important, becoming totally aware of the other person. Such awareness can show itself through mindful:

- movement: becoming aware of how movement and the use of physical space affects human relationships
- speech: recognising the uniqueness and giftedness as well as the concerns and anxieties of the other
- touch: becomes more than purely functional, becoming a vector for reassurance, connectedness and healing.

It is vital for the nurse to be aware of and forge links / bridges with resources such as local faith communities that could be of use to those with a learning disability (Gaventa, 2010). Such links may prove useful in gaining an understanding of faith community-based spiritual identity and practices. Again, such links may be important in encouraging faith community leaders to engage with patients and service users who have a learning disability whilst they are in your care. Nurses who work specifically with those who have a learning disability will also have a role in facilitating and participating in the training of both nursing and medical colleagues and local faith communities and their leaders. Such participation in the training of nursing and medical colleagues and faith communities could include presenting at team meetings, running or being involved in workshops or seminars aimed at nurses or faith community leaders, or presenting at conferences. It may also be useful to submit posters to various conferences that are targeted at nurses and other health and social care professionals.

14.6 Conclusion

Whilst great care must be taken not to impose one's own personal beliefs (because to do so can be seen as abusive), spirituality can often be seen as a very personal, complex, fulfilling yet challenging and confusing way of expressing oneself and one's identity. This is even more so when people have a learning disability, as a result of the differing ways in which they communicate, engage and interact with the world, the environment and the people around them. It is as unethical and unprofessional to ignore, downplay, patronise or belittle the importance of spirituality in the lives of those with a learning disability, as it is to engage with and treat anyone else in like manner.

CHAPTER SUMMARY

Key points to take away from *Chapter 14*:

- ☑ Those with a learning disability have as much right and need to explore, experience and express their spirituality as anyone else.
- ☑ Spirituality has a number of meanings and definitions, with many of these definitions involving a personal search for meaning and purpose in life which may or may not be related to religion.
- ☑ Many of those with a learning disability are likely to experience a number of barriers to a personal experiencing and expression of an authentic spirituality.
- ☑ There are a number of resources that can be of use to those with a learning disability, to nurses or to both.
- ☑ The role of the nurse is to be aware of and understand the importance of spirituality in people's lives and to act appropriately on this awareness and understanding.

Questions

Question 14.1   How would *you* define spirituality and religion? Explain the relationships between the two concepts.

Question 14.2   When helping to support a person's spirituality and religious engagement, what parts of the *NMC Code* will you be meeting, and how?

Question 14.3   Re-read the sections above on resources and the role of the nurse. How would you devise a five-step plan based on these sections that meets the spiritual needs of those with a learning disability?

Question 14.4   How would you assess a person's spiritual and religious needs? What tools would you use and why? What would you assess and why? How would you adapt existing spiritual assessment tools for use by those with a learning disability?

Question 14.5   How would you use the nursing process when supporting the spiritual and/or religious needs of an adult and a child with a learning disability? Is the use of the nursing process relevant and appropriate within this context?

REFERENCES

Barber, C. (2013) Article 6: spirituality and learning disability. *British Journal of Healthcare Assistants*, **7(4)**: 180–5.

Bogdashina, O. (2013) *Autism and Spirituality: psyche, self and spirit in people on the autism spectrum*. Jessica Kingsley Publishers.

Gardner, F. (2011) *Critical spirituality: a holistic approach to contemporary practice*. Routledge.

Gaventa, W. (2010) 'Spirituality issues and strategies'. In Friedman, S. and Helm, D. (eds) *End-of-life Care for Children and Adults with Intellectual and Developmental Disabilities*. American Association on Intellectual and Developmental Disabilities.

Hall, T. and Edwards, K. (2002) The Spiritual Assessment Inventory: a theistic model and measure for assessing spiritual development. *Journal for the Scientific Study of Religion*, **41(2)**: 341–57.

Hays, J., Meador, K., Branch, P. and George, L. (2001) The Spiritual History Scale in four dimensions (SHS-4): validity and reliability. *Gerontologist*, **41(2)**: 239–49.

King, D. (2002) 'Spirituality and medicine'. In Mengel, M., Holleman, W. and Field, S. (eds) *Fundamentals of Clinical Practice: a textbook on the patient, doctor and society*, 2nd edition. Springer.

King, M. and Hunt, R. (1972) Measuring the religious variable: replication. *Journal for the Scientific Study of Religion*, **11(3)**: 240–51.

MacKinlay, E. (2006) *Spiritual Growth and Care in the Fourth Age of Life*. Jessica Kingsley Publishers.

Males, J. and Boswell, C. (1990) Spiritual needs of people with a mental handicap. *Nursing Standard*, **4(48)**: 35–7.

McSherry, W. (2007) *The Meaning of Spirituality and Spiritual Care within Nursing and Health Care Practice*. Quay Books.

Murray, R. and Zentner, J. (1989) *Nursing Concepts for Health Promotion*. Prentice Hall.

NHS (2018) *Mindfulness*. Available at: www.nhs.uk/mental-health/self-help/tips-and-support/mindfulness/ (accessed 4 January 2022).

Puchalski, C. and Romer, L. (2000) Taking a spiritual history allows clinicians to understand patients more fully. *Journal of Palliative Medicine*, **3(1)**: 129–37.

Reed, P. (1992) An emerging paradigm for the investigation of spirituality in nursing. *Research in Nursing and Health*, **15**: 349–57.

Schneiders, S. (1989) Spirituality in the academy. *Theological Studies*, **50**: 678–97.

Stoll, R. (1989) 'The essence of spirituality'. In Carson, V. (ed.) *Spiritual Dimensions of Nursing Practice*. W.B. Saunders.

Sharma, R., Astrow, A., Texeira, K. and Sulmasy, D. (2012) The Spiritual Needs Assessment for Patients (SNAP): development and validation of a comprehensive instrument to assess unmet spiritual needs. *Journal of Pain Symptom Management*, **44(1)**: 44–51.

Swinton, J. (2001) *A Space to Listen: meeting the spiritual needs of people with learning disabilities*. Mental Health Foundation.

Swinton, J. (2002) Spirituality and the lives of people with learning disabilities: a review. *Tizard Learning Disability Review*, **7(4)**: 29–35.

Tanyi, R. (2002) Towards clarification of the meaning of spirituality. *Journal of Advanced Nursing*, **39(5)**: 500–9.

Wiseman, J. (2006) *Spirituality and Mysticism*. Orbis Books.

Wattis, J., Curran, S. and Rogers, M. (2017) 'What does spirituality mean for patients, practitioners and health care organisations?' In Wattis, J., Curran, S. and Rogers, M. (eds) *Spiritually Competent Practice in Health Care*. CRC Press.

Wu, L-F., Koo, M., Liao, Y., Chen, Y. and Yeh, D. (2016) Development and validation of the Spiritual Care Needs Inventory for acute care hospital patients in Taiwan. *Clinical Nurse Research*, **25(6)**: 590–606.

RESOURCES

Books Beyond Words: https://booksbeyondwords.co.uk/ (accessed 4 January 2022)

Faith and Light Communities: www.faithandlight.org.uk (accessed 4 January 2022)

L'Arche: www.larche.org.uk (accessed 4 January 2022)

The Kairos Forum: www.kairosforum.org (accessed 4 January 2022)

Chapter 15
The future and learning disability

AIMS AND LEARNING OUTCOMES

The aims of this chapter are to:

- Summarise a number of the key points that have been made throughout this book

- Highlight the current situation with regard to support and care for those with a learning disability

- Highlight a number of possible future issues regarding such support and care.

By the end of this chapter, you will be:

- Reminded of many of the issues highlighted in previous chapters

- Able to discuss the historical and current position of those with a learning disability with regard to care and support

- Able to discuss possible future issues regarding those with a learning disability and their care and support, and to discuss these issues with those with a learning disability

- Able to discuss historical, current and future issues in learning disability service commissioning, design and provision

- Able to include the contents of such discussions in current and future work with those with a learning disability.

15.1 Introduction

The varied and often complex ways in which those with a learning disability and, where appropriate, those on the autism spectrum seek and express their identities and have their support needs recognised and supported has been the focus of this book. A 'whole life' approach from birth to death has been deliberately adopted in order to counteract the misplaced perception that learning disability is a childhood condition which improves with age. This book has also covered a range of relatively 'difficult' issues such as sexuality, spirituality, ageing, dying and death, discrimination, informal caregiving and those with a learning disability as both crime victim and perpetrator; the intention has been to stimulate thought, discussion and, where appropriate, action. This final chapter will look back over these chapters, placing them within historical contexts if needed, and explore where those with a learning disability and learning disability services are now and where they are likely to be in 10–20 years' time. Part of this discussion will be to explore whether the 'predictive comments' made in the concluding chapter in *Caring for People with Learning Disabilities* have actually come to pass and if not, why not and whether this will have any impact on any future 'predictive comments'.

15.2 Past

The first version of this book, *Caring for People with Learning Disabilities*, was published in February 2015 and I am now writing this final chapter for the new version, *Essentials: Learning Disability*, in February and March 2021 during the Covid-19 pandemic; the book will be published in 2022. Whilst much has remained the same over these seven years in terms of thinking, attitudes, practices, experiences and legislation there has also been much change, some of which has been for the better and some not. This current 'past' would have included the 'present' from the first version of the book.

The definitions and meanings of learning disability outlined in *Chapter 2* were fair and accurate. Such meanings and definitions have not changed over the past six years and are unlikely to change over the coming decade. The assertion made in the 2015 version of the book that "unless one is able to understand what learning disability is, health and social care and support of those with a learning disability will be greatly impoverished" is still valid and has not changed over the intervening six years. Unless one is aware of and understands the past, including historical definitions of learning disability, one is more likely and possibly even 'condemned' to internalise and repeat errors in thinking, attitudes, language and practices to the detriment of those with a learning disability. Whilst good-quality 'basic nursing care' can be offered without such an awareness, an awareness and understanding is essential if more than 'basic nursing care' is to be offered to those with a learning disability and/or those on the autism spectrum.

In a nutshell, the sentiment expressed in the first version that "you as a care professional may wholeheartedly believe that you are giving of your best, I as a patient or service user may perceive and experience a poor or terrible service!" could be a somewhat crude soundbite summary of the 2007 Mencap report *Death by Indifference*. Mencap has produced a number of follow-up reports since this initial 2007 report, all of which have suggested that nurses' knowledge about, attitudes towards and care for those with learning disabilities have not improved. However, many hospitals, GP practices and community health centres are aware of the existence and needs of those with a learning disability and that these needs are both the same as and different from those who do not have a learning disability, and those with a learning disability are being treated more as individuals and less as a large group, and this may be seen as a small improvement. However, the idea that a 'one size fits all' approach still exists, lurking behind the scenes.

Again, the assertion was made in the first version that general / adult registered nurses seem to be more at home with addressing the physical manifestations and meeting the needs of more profound disabilities such as mobility issues, pain management, personal hygiene and dressing, eating, drinking, elimination and breathing. The point was made that the nurse should perhaps be more aware of and understand the whole person behind all these physical health issues. Again, this is still valid and relevant.

Although it is vital to have a basic understanding of the history of learning disability and learning disability care as without such understanding we are condemned to repeat its mistakes, Gilbert (2009) has already done this and to some depth; I did not and do not see the point of repeating him.

The chapter on legislation, law, policy and reports (*Chapter 4*) has been updated in line with developments and changes in law and Government reports. As new Bills enter the statute books and become law and new policies, White and Green Papers, and reports are published, so this chapter will need updating from time to time.

Chapter 5 on caring for those with a learning disability within a general hospital setting perhaps forms the centre of both versions of this book, as possibly most of those who will buy and read it are likely to be working within an acute general hospital. Given that, a much slimmer book that focuses purely on providing and celebrating good-quality nursing care to those with a learning disability and autism spectrum conditions in these settings rather than a more general book such as this, might be helpful. However, *Chapter 5* (and, indeed, the whole of this revised version) does highlight a range of excellent work that is being carried out by nurses in hospital care settings such as the use of hospital 'passports', access to further training and development, and the improved care experienced by those with a learning disability from pre-admittance visits to post-discharge follow up. It was the intention that positive as well as negative aspects of care as experienced by those with a learning disability would be promoted.

Issues around sexuality, old age, death, and spirituality (*Chapters 9–11* and *14*, respectively) have faced a range of responses from many care professionals including being historically ignored, paid lip service to and in some incidences ridiculed. Whilst a lack of awareness and understanding of these issues may have contributed to this range of responses, attitudes, and resultant possible poor practice, ultimately these responses cannot be justified and they are likely to place the nurse in breach of the NMC *Code*. Despite increasing media attention being given to those with a learning disability and increasing self-advocacy it is unlikely that this has changed over the past six years. These are important although very difficult issues to get to grips with and are likely to have profound effects on all of us – sexuality and spirituality have such a major impact on our identity as human beings and yet strangely tend to be forgotten or at the very least downplayed by many who work with or write about those with a learning disability. Such omissions by other people tend to make lives more marginalised and poorer. It was the intention within these chapters to highlight some of these issues and promote the good work that many nurses are engaged in, in the areas of sexuality, ageing, dying, death and bereavement, and spirituality.

Chapter 12 on 'informal' caregivers was marked with considerable anger on the part of many caregivers and this was deliberate, as it would have been only too easy to 'look the other way', to 'brush the issues under the carpet' by claiming that caregivers do not experience significant difficulties in their caring responsibilities at the hands of care professionals. Whilst there are many good examples of care professionals 'getting it right' and 'going the extra mile' with regard to support for caregivers, these are heavily outnumbered by indifferent or poor care and support which will have an impact on the physical and mental health of the caregiver. Unfortunately, this has not changed since the 2015 version of this book and may have actually got worse over the years despite the input of and campaigning by carer organisations such as Carers UK.

I stand by my decision not to 'airbrush' this frustration and pain out of the text. To have done so neither respects caregivers nor is it likely to bring about change. Likewise, with *Chapter 13* on disability discrimination; no one is served well by trying to deny that disability discrimination exists and can have a profound effect on individuals, care professionals and society. Indeed, Saba Salman, a journalist who has a sister with a learning disability, made this point during an interview on BBC Radio 4's *World at One* news and current affairs programme on Thursday 4th February 2021 (time slot: 13:22–13:28).

However, it is my intention and hope that by including this material that some readers may see as portraying a negative picture which they may not recognise in their own clinical area of practice, readers will be helped to understand the necessity for improvement and how they can improve their own practice. The idea is to challenge and change systemic and individual failings into success stories and in so doing, ensure that disability and carer discrimination will be 'consigned to the dustbin of history'.

15.3 Present

It must be kept in mind here that this current 'present' would have been the 'future' in *Caring for People with Learning Disabilities*. There have been many positive changes in the lives of those with a learning disability, although these have been more by 'evolution' rather than 'revolution'.

There has been a greater understanding of those with a learning disability and their needs on the part of the non-learning disability specialist, an understanding that is matched by perhaps a slower and more gradual evolution rather than revolution in terms of changes in service delivery. That is not to say that changes in awareness, understanding and service delivery did not happen, as clearly they did and I hope that this small book would have played a tiny part in that change. Those with a learning disability are more involved in the teaching and training of health and social care staff through presenting at conferences, teaching nursing students or running workshops. There has been a consultation document in early 2019 that resulted in a call for all health and social care professionals to receive ongoing training in learning disability and autism. However, given the current Covid-19 pandemic, it is debatable as to the reality of the planning and existence of such training: has professional development in learning disability and autism issues been 'kicked into the long grass' due to current health problems and priorities?

There are many areas of the UK that have learning disability, autism and mental health partnership boards which do have quite powerful self-advocacy input and these partnership boards come into their own when feeding into and implementing local, regional and national initiatives, strategies and services. However, for these boards to work well it needs to be a genuine partnership rather than window dressing and needs to be led by people with a learning disability or those on the autism spectrum.

The suggestion was made in the first version of this book that a national service framework (NSF) for those with learning disabilities that sets out both the general and more specific directions for service commissioning and delivery at national, regional and local levels was needed. This has still not been actioned and at the moment, learning disability is one of the conditions that does not have such a framework, although the NSF for long-term conditions is perhaps the best fit in terms of appropriateness. This still needs to be followed by a law that focuses specifically on learning disability, particularly in adults, in much the same way as the Autism Act 2009 did for adults on the autism spectrum. At the moment, the Autism Act is the only disability-specific law that exists in the UK.

However, disability discrimination, be it overt or covert, deliberate or accidental still exists in terms of:
- poor access to or take-up of the vaccine for Covid-19
- the way that those with a learning disability are cared for and treated within healthcare settings (see the Saba Salman citation above)
- the imposition of 'do not attempt cardiopulmonary resuscitation' (DNACPR) orders purely on the grounds of a person having a learning disability and without the person being consulted or having their views taken into account (Learning Disability England, 2020).

Whilst these issues should be dealt with through appropriate ongoing professional development opportunities, current health problems and priorities and staff exhaustion may lead to a decline in the availability or uptake of such opportunities. And whilst the availability and uptake of good quality professional development should not be seen as the 'silver bullet' in terms of eradicating poor quality or less than ethical care, it will go a long way to addressing underlying care attitudes, issues and practices.

15.4 **Future**

In the first version of this book, four questions were asked, questions which are still valid: where do you see, and where would you *like* to see those with a learning disability in, say, twenty years' time? Where do you see, and where would you *like* to see learning disability *services* in twenty years' time? It must be kept in mind that there is a world of difference between 'where you see' and 'where you *would like to see*'. The former is much more likely to be realistic, pragmatic and even slightly pessimistic in tone, whereas the latter is tending towards the aspirational.

Where do you see those with a learning disability? It is likely that those with a learning disability will be more involved in the teaching and training of health and social care staff through presenting at conferences, teaching nursing students or running workshops. However, it is also likely that those with a learning disability will still face discrimination and poor quality of care and support, be these accidental or intentional. As long as people who espouse similar views to Collin Brewer and Nick Martin (see *Chapter 13*) are in positions of influence, there will also be people and institutions that will openly and deliberately discriminate. After the BBC *Panorama* TV programme that highlighted the abuse at Winterbourne View in November 2011, service commissioners, designers and providers said, 'never again'. However, it was held by some of those with a learning disability and disability advocates and activists that Winterbourne View was just the tip of the iceberg and that there were many other 'Winterbourne Views' out there. Events have since proved this to be correct in the form of Whorlton Hall in 2019 and Cawston Park in 2021. Have service commissioners, designers and providers, have politicians listened, understood and learnt any long-lasting lessons? Could Winterbourne View and Whorlton Hall happen again? That is debatable!

Where would you like to see those with learning disabilities? In an ideal world, those with a learning disability will be fully engaged in service commissioning, design and delivery. There are a range of platforms that are available for those with a learning disability and/or autism to be so engaged. Those with a learning disability are increasingly used as 'mystery shoppers' and assessors of services, or sit on interview panels or are involved in the interview processes for registered nurses or nursing academics. A number of voluntary sector organisations are actively encouraging those with a learning disability and/or autism spectrum conditions to become fully involved in the running of that organisation through becoming trustees. Many regions within the UK will have learning disability or autism partnership boards, with these boards being co-chaired by people with a learning disability and/or autism and those with a learning disability are seen and valued as members equal to service commissioners and providers. Such opportunities have been brought about through greater self-advocacy and political awareness and clout and can only expand and develop in the future.

Where would you like to see learning disability services in years to come? Again, in an ideal world, health and social care, acute (hospital), community and residential care and support services communicating and cooperating with each other in the commissioning, design and delivery of services. If a person with a learning disability is admitted to hospital for any reason, discharge assessment and planning is done properly, holistically and is person-centred. All too often, discharge planning fails due to poor communication and cooperation between service providers, the person with a learning disability and, where appropriate, their families. People do not 'sing from the same hymn sheet', resulting in poor, inadequate, inappropriate or in some cases a lack of services being offered to those with a learning disability. Those with a learning disability will be looking more at a far greater understanding of those with a learning disability and their needs on the part of the non-learning disability specialist, an understanding that is matched by perhaps a slower and more gradual evolution rather than revolution in terms of changes in service delivery.

There is a need for a national service framework (NSF) for those with learning disabilities that sets out both the general and more specific directions for service commissioning and delivery at national, regional and local levels. At the moment, as it was in 2015 when the first version of this book was published, learning disability is one of the conditions that does not have such a framework, although the NSF for 'long-term conditions' is perhaps the 'best fit' in terms of appropriateness. This could perhaps be followed by a law that focuses specifically on learning disability, particularly in adults, in much the same way as the Autism Act 2009 did for adults on the autism spectrum. At the moment, the Autism Act is the only disability-specific law that we have. There is also a need for those with a learning disability to self-advocate in terms of being actively involved in contributing to both any NSFs and legislation. However, this may involve a massive redistribution of power from existing politicians, service designers and commissioners.

Where do you see learning disability services in years to come? The answer to this question depends on a range of political and economic issues, priorities and agendas. There is likely to be much greater interdisciplinary and multi-professional training at both undergraduate and postgraduate levels. Such interdisciplinary training and networking is already happening but it needs to improve. Those with a learning disability will be heavily involved in facilitating and leading such training and networks. It is likely that high-quality interdisciplinary training would lead to genuine 'joined-up' thinking, communication and working between health and social care and support commissioners, designers and providers, training which will be led by those with a learning disability. Holistic and multidisciplinary care and support assessments, planning, implementation and evaluation, where the person with a learning disability is at the centre rather than the periphery and is fully involved rather than being a passive recipient of this process, will be the norm. Having said that, it is likely that some of the barriers to such holistic communication and working including different agendas and priorities, different 'power structures', 'professional politics', professional accountability, management structures and different ways of working will continue, to the detriment of service users.

In-service training and professional development will be a major issue over the coming years, due in part to the accumulation of health and social care scandals and associated reports such as Mencap's *Death by Indifference*, Winterbourne View,

Whorlton Hall and Cawston Park and in part to the planned introduction of the mandatory three-tier training system (see *Chapter 1*). The level of training that is engaged in will be determined by the role and extent and type of contact that individual health and social care staff have with people with learning disabilities and/or autism. The quality and content of such training may vary depending on the skills, knowledge and experience of training providers and how much money service providers are willing (and able) to invest in such training and the value that they place on professional development. The old adage that 'you can lead a horse to water but you cannot make it drink' may be relevant here but it is to be hoped that training and professional development will have a positive impact on attitudes and practices in caring for people with learning disabilities.

However, much of this admittedly 'crystal ball gazing' into the future depends on the will of politicians and service commissioners, designers and providers to make positive changes and this in turn depends on people's ability and willingness to share power. Where this ability and willingness is not evident, any 'positive changes' regarding service design and delivery systems will be mere 'window dressing' and are unlikely to impress anyone, least of all those with a learning disability and/or autism spectrum condition or their families. This may sound harsh but ask yourselves two groups of questions:

1. Why, despite the universal condemnation of the 'care' experienced at Winterbourne View, did some consider Winterbourne View to be just the 'tip of the iceberg'? Why did very few people foresee the possibility of a similar scandal happening again and prevent it? Why did we have a Whorlton Hall? Has anyone learnt the lessons from these or will we in another few years face a similar scandal with the predictable shock and horror? Will those with power and authority do everything that they can and more to prevent it? If not, why not?

2. Why, despite the presence of voluntary sector organisations whose role it is to safeguard, protect and be a voice for those with a learning disability and/ or autism, were many of those with a learning disability denied the Covid-19 vaccine? Why was it that it took journalists, many of whom had close relatives with a learning disability, rather than these voluntary sector organisations to successfully campaign for all those with a learning disability to receive the vaccine? Given that the same applies to DNACPR 'orders', did those with power and authority abdicate their role and duty to act forcefully as advocates? If so, why were and are they allowed to 'get away with it'?

To change tack a bit, the value, purpose and very existence of registered learning disability nurses have been debated over many years and even decades and will continue to be debated over many years and decades to come. Various published reports have called into question the purpose and value of continuing with the four-branch entry into nursing (adult, children, mental health and learning disability). The recommendation was made a few years ago to restructure pre-registration nurse training and suggested having a single-branch generalist / adult training where all students will graduate and register *as a nurse* and will have enough basic knowledge and skills to work in any clinical setting and with any patient or service user group. Those who want to specialise and work with those who have a mental health issue, those who have a learning disability, or children will have to engage in further postgraduate / post-registration training in much the same way as medical doctors do. Whilst there may on the surface be some merit to such a suggestion, the questions have to be asked: will there be an appetite for further, in-depth and expensive post-registration training, given that many if not most newly registered nurses may not be in a financially strong enough position to engage in such further training or have the energy to do so? Will this lead to a diminution of knowledge and skills within the nursing workforce, a diminution that will inevitably and negatively affect the quality of care that those with a learning disability will receive and a diminution that could pave the way for further Winterbourne View or Whorlton Hall type scandals? Again, it is worth citing from the first version of this book:

> "I fear, in that case, that we will return to the old institutions where choice, dignity and respect did not exist. Those who lived in these old hospitals still tell me of bath times when three service users were being bathed at the same time and in the same bath room: one getting undressed, one being bathed and one getting dried and dressed again. It would mean going back to a time when everyone got hot tea which was served in huge metal tea pots with milk and loads of sugar already added, whether people liked tea or not, whether they liked sugar with their tea or not. There was no choice."

That was a reality that many would wish to downplay and say that we have moved on from. However, if there is a single nurse registration, could we return to such a situation cited above due to a lack of learning disability nurses, and adult trained nurses not having the necessary skills, knowledge and experience in learning disability care?

Student learning disability nurses are still being faced with a lack of understanding and acceptance by many nurses who are not learning disability trained. *"Well, you are not really nurses are you"* and *"What you are doing is not real nursing"* are still comments that are repeated mantra-like by many adult / general trained nurses during student clinical placements. Such comments as these are even repeated by some in senior management and academic positions, all of whom should know better. However, if those with a learning disability and those who are on the autism spectrum can be seen as simply a 'natural variant of the human condition', as part of the rich diversity of what it means to be human, do we still need specialist healthcare services for those with a learning disability, nursing or otherwise? After all, such services can be quite expensive and in a very cash-strapped health and social care environment, priorities have to be set and decisions made based on these priorities, and sometimes those with a learning disability have been viewed as having a relatively low priority. Whilst these and similar sentiments may have some traction within healthcare commissioning, funding and delivery (and please note that this is not the same as me agreeing with these sentiments), they are only so to an extent. Priorities *do* have to be set that meet both the requirements of individuals and local, regional and national communities and the constraints of budgets. There is no such thing as a 'money tree' or a bottomless 'money pit'; there is not an endless supply of money and other resources and sometimes unpalatable decisions that may be viewed by some as unfair and unjust have to be made: for some people, groups and communities to receive optimum health and social care, others have to lose out. That is a reality that is often hard to accept but that is a reality nonetheless.

It could be argued that the answer to both major sets of questions above lies partly in our ability and responsibility as nurses, both individually and collectively, to say 'enough', 'not on our watch'. The future lies in our hands so let us not squander these opportunities.

15.5 Conclusion

Looking back, whether it is over the course of a book such as this one or over a period of time, say the seven years between publication of the two versions of a book such as this one, is relatively easy to do: hindsight is a wonderful thing! Being asked to produce a revised version of a book allows the author the opportunity to review both the contents of the original and put right any errors or omissions that have been found – and there have been a few. Looking forward into a crystal ball and predicting with any accuracy not only potential events but their potential consequences for those with a learning disability has always been hazardous. For example, it could not have been predicted with any certainty in 2013–14 when I wrote this chapter for *Caring for People with Learning Disabilities* that there would have been a 're-run' of Winterbourne View and that nothing would have been learnt in the intervening years, and yet we had Whorlton Hall a few years later.

The next decade for those with a learning disability (and those on the autism spectrum such as myself) looks interesting to say the least. That decade in terms of life events and consequences and health and social care for those with a learning disability rests in all of our hands. A lack of knowledge on the part of health and social care providers and professionals must never become the norm, as to allow it to do so harms the individual person with a learning disability, their families, care professionals and society at large. To allow this to happen betrays the trust that those with a learning disability have in care professionals. The future is yours, so make it happen and make it a good one.

REFERENCES

Gilbert, T. (2009) 'From the workhouse to citizenship: four ages of learning disability'. In Jukes, M. (ed.) *Learning Disability Nursing Practice*. Quay Books.

Learning Disability England (2020) *Disabled People's Rights, DNAR and Covid19*. Available at: www.learningdisabilityengland.org.uk/coronavirus-hub/other-resources-that-can-help/disabled-peoples-rights-dnar-and-covid19/ (accessed 4 January 2022).

Glossary

AS: Asperger's syndrome; the 'higher IQ' end of the autism spectrum.

ASC: Autism spectrum condition, ranging from 'classic autism' (a triad of impairments in social interaction, social communication and the use of language, and in limited social imagination as reflected in restricted, repetitive and stereotyped patterns of behaviour and activities) through to Asperger's syndrome. There are about 670 000 people in the UK (about 1.1% of the UK population) who are known to be on the autism spectrum.

ASD: Autism spectrum disorder. ASD and ASC are often used interchangeably. Some people prefer the term 'condition' whilst others use 'disorder'.

AS/HFA: Asperger's syndrome / high-functioning autism.

Developmental delay: The term that is currently used in the USA to designate those with a learning disability. This has largely taken over from the term 'mental retardation' (The American Association on Mental Retardation continued to use the term 'mental retardation' until 2006).

Down's syndrome: Down's syndrome is a genetic condition caused by the presence of an extra chromosome in the body's cells. Down's syndrome is not a disease, and it is not a hereditary condition. It occurs by chance at conception. Everyone with Down's syndrome will have some degree of learning disability. Certain physical characteristics and health conditions are common among people with Down's syndrome. Down's syndrome used to be called 'mongolism'.

Epilepsy: Epilepsy is a neurological condition which affects around 600 000 people in the UK (1% of the UK population) where there is a tendency to experience recurrent seizures (fits), of which there are around 40 different types. Epilepsy can affect anyone, from any walk of life and from any age. For more information see: www.epilepsy.org.uk/press/facts.

Learning disability:
- An arrested or incomplete development of mind
- A significantly reduced ability to understand new or complex information (impaired intelligence and cognitive functioning)
- A significantly reduced ability to learn new skills (impaired intelligence and cognitive functioning), with

- A reduced ability to cope independently (impaired social functioning) and
- Which started before adulthood and with a lasting effect on development.

Mencap: A voluntary sector organisation that raises the profile of, and campaigns for those with a learning disability and their families. Its services are UK-wide.

Mental handicap: An older term used to designate those with a learning disability that was used throughout the 1980s and early 1990s.

Mental retardation: An older term used to designate those with a learning disability that was used throughout the 1960s.

Mental subnormality: An older term used to designate those with a learning disability that was used throughout the 1970s.

Nurse: A nurse is a person who has successfully undergone three years of training and preparation, usually at undergraduate / first-degree level, and is registered with and regulated by the Nursing and Midwifery Council (NMC). Other countries are likely to have similar training and registration requirements. This is distinct from health or social care assistants or nursing assistants / auxiliaries who do not embark upon or complete nurse training and, at the moment, are not professionally registered and regulated.

Nursing Associate: A person who has completed a foundation degree in nursing and healthcare and whose role is registered and regulated by the NMC. Such a person will carry out many of the roles of the registered nurse but under the supervision of the registered nurse.

RN(LD): Registered nurse (learning disability): the current learning disability nurse qualification and NMC entry.

RN(MH): Registered nurse (mental handicap): an older learning disability nurse qualification used throughout the 1980s.

RN(MS): Registered nurse (mental subnormality): an older learning disability nurse qualification used throughout the 1970s.

Resources

BILD: British Institute of Learning Disability. BILD uses its books and journals, conferences and events, and membership information and networks to encourage the exchange of new ideas and good practice. BILD also provides consultancy and, through support for the health and social care qualifications and training in the workplace, can help support the development of staff and the organisations they work for. Its website is: www.bild.org.uk

Carers Trust: One of the two main voluntary sector organisations specifically for 'informal caregivers'. This charity campaigns and offers advice, information and support for informal carers and care professionals. Its website is: www.carers.org

Carers UK: One of the two main voluntary sector organisations specifically for 'informal caregivers'. Carers UK provides a wide range of information for both caregivers and care professionals, runs caregiver support groups throughout the UK, and campaigns on caregiver issues locally, regionally and nationally. Its website is: www.carersuk.org

Cerebra: Founded in 2001, Cerebra is a unique national charity that strives to improve the lives of children with brain-related neurological conditions such as learning disability and autism spectrum conditions, through research, education and direct, ongoing support. Its website is: www.cerebra.org.uk

Down's Syndrome Association: Provides information and support on all aspects of Down's syndrome to all who require it. Its website is: www.downs-syndrome.org.uk

(Information regarding a number of other forms of learning disability such as Rett syndrome and tuberous sclerosis can also be found on the internet).

Houses of Parliament all-party interest group on learning disability: This is a group of MPs and peers who have a special interest in learning disability issues. Its website is: www.publications.parliament.uk/pa/cm/cmallparty/register/learning-disability.htm

Kairos: Kairos was established by John Swinton (professor of practical theology at the University of Aberdeen) and Cristina Gangemi to provide advice, information, advocacy and support for individuals who have a learning disability and their families regarding spirituality, religious practice and the vital role they have within communities. The creation of a space for the development of networks of lay people, professionals and religious communities was seen as crucial as a way of providing information regarding spirituality and learning disability. Its website is: www. kairosforum.org

KIDS: KIDS is a UK voluntary sector organisation which, in its 40-year history, has pioneered a number of approaches and programmes for children and young people who have a disability. These include home learning (Portage), parent partnerships, adventure playgrounds and the inclusion of children with disabilities in mainstream settings. Its website is: www.kids.org.uk

L'Arche: In a world that places such value on success and winning, L'Arche communities are places where people can take time to explore who they are, not just what they can do. They are places of welcome where people are transformed by an intense experience of community, relationship, disability and difference. Set up by the now disgraced Jean Vanier (see *Chapter 14*), L'Arche is an international voluntary sector organisation that provides residential services for those with a learning disability along broadly Christian lines. Although Vanier is disgraced, it must be pointed out that L'Arche is not. Its website is: www.larche.org.uk

Learning disability liaison nurses: Learning disability liaison nurses (LDLNs) are specialist learning disability nurses who are increasingly based in general/acute hospitals. Their main roles include:

- working in collaboration with the acute hospital to enable open and easy access to healthcare services for people with learning disabilities
- being a point of contact and resource for the non-learning disability specialist
- working at a strategic level with health professionals, managers and commissioners to achieve the health agenda of the White Paper *Valuing People*.

They can be contacted via the hospital switchboard.

Learning Disability Practice: A monthly peer-reviewed journal from the publishing arm of the Royal College of Nursing (RCN Publishing); it can be viewed on its website: https://journals.rcni.com/learning-disability-practice

Mencap: Mencap is one of the main voluntary sector organisations that campaigns for those with a learning disability and provides support, information and advocacy for those with a learning disability, their families and care professionals nationally, regionally and locally. Its website is: www.mencap.org.uk

Mind: Mind is one of a wide range of voluntary sector organisations that provide information and support, and campaign for those who experience mental health issues, their families and care professionals. Its website is: www.mind.org.uk

Naidex: Naidex National is the home of the UK independent living market. It is the largest UK exhibition and conference of its kind, showcasing a comprehensive range of products, services and workshops / seminars that enable people with a disability to live more independently. Naidex takes place each year at the NEC, Birmingham. Its website is: www.naidex.co.uk

National Autistic Society (NAS): One of the main organisations that raises the profile of and campaigns for those on the autism spectrum and provides information about autism spectrum conditions for those on the spectrum, their families and care professionals. Its council and trustee board includes those who are on the autism spectrum. Its website is: www.autism.org.uk

Reports on learning disability care: There have been a large number of official reports into the care of those with a learning disability over the past 40 years. See *Chapter 4* for a list of these.

Scope: Scope is a national voluntary sector organisation that raises the profile of people with disabilities through providing information, campaigning and offering a range of services for children and adults with disabilities; it is primarily focused on those with complex support needs. Its website is: www.scope.org.uk

Support groups: There are a wide variety of support groups for those with a learning disability, their parents and their siblings. At the moment, whether there are any support groups specifically for children of those with a learning disability is unknown. In the first instance, contact your local or regional Mencap branch / office or the hospital's learning disability liaison nurse for advice and possible contact details.

UK legislation: Information regarding a wide range of UK laws / legislation, Parliamentary Bills, White Papers and related issues can be found at the UK Government's website: www.legislation.gov.uk

Examples of such legislation include:
- The Mental Capacity Act 2005: www.legislation.gov.uk/ukpga/2005/9/contents
- The Autism Act 2009: www.legislation.gov.uk/ukpga/2009/15/contents
- The Equality Act 2010: www.legislation.gov.uk/ukpga/2010/15/contents

Index

If you wish to follow the views/thoughts of the individuals who appear in this book, their names are in speech marks in the index